ABC OF WORK RELATED DISORDERS

ABC OF WORK RELATED DISORDERS

Edited by

DAVID SNASHALL

Clinical Director, Occupational Health Department, Guy's and St Thomas's Hospital NHS Trust, Lambeth Palace Road, London

BMJ
Publishing
Group

© BMJ Publishing Group 1997

First published in 1997
by the BMJ Publishing Group, BMA House, Tavistock Square,
London WC1H 9JR

British Library Cataloguing in Publication Data

A catalogue record for this book is available from the British Library

ISBN 0-7279-1154-6

Cover illustration by Jeanne Berg, © The Stock Illustration Source.

Typset by Apek Typesetters, Nailsea, Bristol.
Printed and bound by Craft Print, Singapore

Contents

Contributors

Anil Adisesh
clinical lecturer
Centre for Occupational Health, University of Manchester, Stopford Building, Manchester

P H Appleby
divisional director
Building Health and Safety, Thorburn Colquhoun, London

Rob B Briner
lecturer
Department of Organisational Psychology, Birkbeck College, University of London, London

David Coggon
reader in occupational and environmental medicine
MRC Environmental Epidemiology Unit, Southampton General Hospital, Southampton

Martyn J F Davidson
head of Medical Service
John Lewis Partnership, London

William W Davies
consultant occupational physician
South Wales Fire and Local Authorities Occupational Health Service, Pontyclun, Wales

Mats Hagberg
professor of work and environmental physiology
National Institute for Working Life, Department of Ergonomics, Epidemiology and Biomechanics, Solna, Sweden

Malcolm I V Jayson
emeritus professor of rheumatology
Rheumatic Diseases Centre, Clinical Sciences Building, Hope Hospital, Salford, Manchester

C M Jones
senior medical officer
Aldwarke Occupational Health Department, British Steel Engineering Steels, Rotherham Works, Rotherham, South Yorkshire

Laila H Kapadia
occupational health physician
Marks and Spencer plc, London

Ira Madan
consultant occupational physician
Occupational Health and Safety Department, Southmead Health Service NHS Trust, Southmead Hospital, Westbury on Trym, Bristol

Julia von Onciul
human resources development manager
LucasVarity plc Group Management, Development and Training, Solihull, West Midlands

Keith Palmer
consultant occupational physician
MRC Environmental Epidemiology Unit, Southampton General Hospital, Southampton

Gordon Parker
head of health and safety services
Centre for Occupational Health, University of Manchester, Stopford Building, Manchester

David Snashall
clinical director
Occupational Health Department, Guy's and St Thomas's Hospital NHS Trust, London

Charles Veys
senior research fellow in occupational medicine
Industrial and Community Health Research Centre, School of Postgraduate Medicine, University of Keele, Staffordshire

Ian R White
consultant dermatologist
St John's Institute of Dermatology, St Thomas's Hospital, London

Preface

Although work is generally considered to be good for your health and a healthy working population is essential to a country's economic and social development, certain kinds of work can be damaging. This book covers the common work related disorders which, although studied and managed by occupational physicians, frequently present to the general practitioner or doctor in the accident and emergency department.

Work patterns are changing, leading to the demise of some of the older occupational diseases such as pneumoconiosis and an increasing recognition of newer conditions, such as occupational asthma, building related disorders and work induced psychological stress. This is not true everywhere, especially in countries where rapid industrial development is occurring. Traditional occupational diseases such as pesticide poisoning and asbestosis are still depressingly common in the developing world. All occupational disease is preventable.

This book will be useful for students of occupational health and occupational hygiene, students of environmental health and doctors of all types who wish to recognise and manage work related conditions successfully. The emphasis is on practical management.

In addition there are chapters for the doctor who wishes to extend a little into occupational health practice—for example on how to do a workplace survey, how to assess fitness for work and, most importantly, how to work with an occupational health department in managing work related disorders. There are also two chapters about the effect of work related disorders, namely chapter 2 on absence from work, and chapter 16 on the legal framework and control of health and safety in Great Britain.

D. Snashall

1 HAZARDS OF WORK

David Snashall

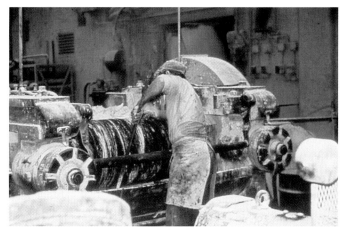

Most readers of this series will consider themselves lucky to have an interesting job. However tedious others may find it, work defines a person—which is one reason why most people who lack the opportunity to work feel disenfranchised. As well as determining our standard of living, work takes up about a third of our waking time, widens our social network, constrains where we can live, and conditions our personalities. "Good" work is life enhancing, but bad working conditions damage your health.

Occupational disorders in general practice

How occupational diseases present in general practice	
Musculoskeletal problems	48%
Respiratory problems	10%
Psychological problems	10%

General practitioners are likely to see as much work induced illness as doctors who work in occupational medicine, who spend most of their time assessing fitness for work or on preventive programmes. Such illnesses do not necessarily present at work, and, as only a minority of workers have access to an occupational health department, they usually first consult their general practitioner.

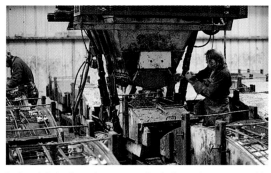

These days few doctors see classic occupational diseases such as pneumoconiosis, heavy metal poisoning, or the various forms of occupational cancer. However, several conditions commonly seen in general practice may be occupational in origin—such as back pain, dermatitis, deafness, and asthma. Many of the injuries sustained at work will also be seen and dealt with in general practice or in accident and emergency departments.

Industrial deafness is easy to miss in its early stages and is not amenable to treatment, but it is wholly preventable.

Reporting occupational illnesses

Surveys in Finland, where reporting is assiduous, have shown rates of occupational disease to be underestimated 3-5 times

Occupational diseases are supposed to be reported to the Health and Safety Executive by employers (usually advised by doctors) under RIDDOR (Reporting of Injuries, Diseases, and Dangerous Occurrences Regulations), but this cannot be relied on—if these official statistics were the only source of information, occupational illness would seem to be very rare.

It has been estimated that 4% of cancer deaths in the United States are directly due to occupational causes. Industrial agents that cause cancer include aromatic amines (rubber and dye industries), asbestos, benzene, ionising radiation, nickel, polyaromatic hydrocarbons, and wood dust

When the 1990 Labour Force Survey asked workers themselves it found that 2·2 million people had had an illness that year which they thought was caused or made worse by their work. It was estimated that these illnesses led to 7% of all general practice consultations. Further cases of occupational disease come to light via the Department of Social Security's compensation scheme for diseases prescribed under the Industrial Injuries Provisions of the Social Security Act 1975.

Total cost of work related illness, injury, and other accidents was £6bn–£12bn (1–2% of gross domestic product) in 1990

Newer initiatives have enabled us to gain a much better picture of certain occupational diseases—notably the SWORD (Surveillance of Work Related and Occupational Respiratory Disease in the United Kingdom) and EPI-DERM reporting systems, which have collected data on respiratory and skin conditions respectively from general practitioners and specialists. These have now been supplemented by OPRA (Occupational Physicians Reporting Activity), which will include other occupational diseases.

Industrial injuries are reported more fully than occupational diseases despite the fact that their impact on workers' health is less. Their cause is usually obvious and recent, whereas cause and effect in occupational disease can be far from obvious and the exposure to the hazardous material may have occurred many years before.

Is an illness occupational?

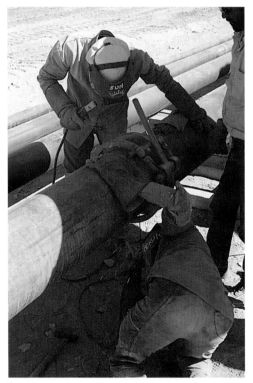

Is lobar pneumonia an occupational disease of welders? Coggon *et al* found that 55 welders had died from lobar pneumonia in recent years against an expected number of 21 (*Lancet* 1994; **344**: 41–3).

Whereas asbestosis and chronic lead poisoning can hardly be described as anything other than occupational diseases (about 70 of these are listed by the Department of Social Security), this may not be true of conditions such as back pain in a construction worker or an upper limb disorder in a keyboard operator when activities outside work may be contributing. A lifetime working in a dusty atmosphere may not lead to chronic bronchitis and emphysema, but, when it is combined with cigarette smoking, it makes this outcome much more likely. Common conditions for which occupational exposure is an important but not the sole or even the major cause can be more reasonably termed work related disease rather than occupational disease.

Certain occupations carry a substantial risk of premature death while others are associated with the likelihood of living a long and healthy life. This is reflected in very different standardised mortality ratios for different jobs, but not all the differences are due to the various hazards of different occupations. Selection factors are important, and social class has an effect (although this is defined by occupation). Non-occupational causes related to behaviour and lifestyle may also be important.

Occupations asociated with high and low standardised mortality ratios (all causes) 1979–83

Occupation	Mortality ratio
Tailors and dressmakers (single women)	194
Road surfacers (men)	165
Bus conductors (men)	150
All occupations (men and single women)	100
Medical practitioners (men)	66
Physical and geological scientists and mathematicians (men)	38
University academic staff (single women)	35

Presentation of work related illnesses

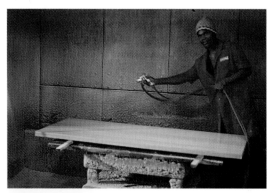

Exposure to solvents at work may be the cause of erratic behaviour at home.

Diseases and conditions of occupational origin usually present in an identical form to the same diseases and conditions due to other factors. Thus, bronchial carcinoma has the same histological appearance and follows the same course whether it results from working with asbestos, uranium mining, or cigarette smoking.

The possibility that a condition is work induced may become apparent only when specific questions are asked because the occupational origin of a disease is usually discovered (and it is discovered only if it is suspected) by the presence of an unusual pattern. For example, in occupational dermatitis the distribution of the lesions may be characteristic. A particular history may be another clue: asthma of late onset is more commonly occupational in origin than asthma that starts early in life. Daytime drowsiness in a fit young factory worker may not be due to late nights and heavy alcohol consumption, but to unsuspected exposure to solvents at work.

An "engineer" may work directly with machinery and risk damage to limbs, skin, and hearing or may spend all day working at a computer and risk back pain, upper limb disorders, and sedentary stress

How to take an occupational history

Question 1
What is your job? or
What do you do for a living?

Question 2
What do you work with? or
What is a typical working day for you? or
What do you actually do at work?

Question 3
How long have you been doing this kind of work?
Have you done any different kinds of work in the past?

Question 4
Have you been told that anything you use at work may make you ill? Has anybody at work had the same symptoms?

Question 5
Do you have any hobbies, like do-it-yourself or gardening, that may bring you into contact with chemicals?

Question 6
Is there an occupational health doctor or nurse at your workplace who I could speak to?

The occupational connection with a condition may not be immediately obvious because patients may give vague answers when asked what their job is. Answers such as "driver," "fitter," or "model" are not very useful, and the closer a doctor can get to extracting a precise job description the better. Sometimes patients will actually have been told (or should have been told) that there are specific hazards associated with their job, or they may know that fellow workers have experienced similar symptoms.

Timing of events

The timing of symptoms is important as they may be related to exposure events during work. Asthma provides a good example of this: many people suffering from occupational asthma develop symptoms only after a delay of some hours, and the condition may present as nocturnal wheeze. It is essential to ask whether symptoms occur during the performance of a specific task and if they occur solely on work days, improving during weekends and holidays.

Working conditions

Patients should be asked specifically about their working conditions. Common problems are dim lighting, noisy machinery, bad office layout, dusty atmosphere, draconian management, and bad morale. Such questioning not only investigates possibilities but gives the doctor a good idea of the general state of a patient's working environment and how he or she reacts to it. A visit to a patient's workplace, if it can be arranged, may be a revelation and just as valuable as a home visit if you want to understand how a patient's health is conditioned and how it might be improved. Knowing about somebody's work can help you to place the person in context and to gain insight. Patients are often happy to talk about the details of their work: this may be less threatening than talking about details of their home life and can promote a better doctor-patient relationship.

The causes of occupational disease can extend beyond the workplace to affect local populations by air or soil pollution and other members of workers' families when overalls soiled with toxic materials are taken home to be washed.

Changing trends in work related illnesses

Trends since 1980 in new cases of occupational disease that justify disability benefit

Decreasing	*Increasing*
Pneumoconiosis	Mesothelioma and asbestosis
Dermatitis	Occupational asthma
Tenosynovitis and beat conditions	Occupational deafness
Tuberculosis and hepatitis	Hand-arm vibration syndrome
Leptospirosis and other infections	

Changes in working practices in Britain are giving rise to work that is more intense and stressful but also less physically demanding. There are more jobs in service industries, more working from home, more handling of newly developed products, and more women at work. This is not necessarily so in many developing countries, where headlong industrialisation has led to sweatshop labour and where occupational accidents and diseases, both acute and chronic, are much more common. As important, of course, are the effects on health of an increasing rate of long term unemployment among the potential workers of the post-industrial world.

Key references
- WHO. *Identification and control of work related diseases.* Geneva: WHO, 1985. (Technical report No 174.)
- Central Statistical Office. *Annual abstract of statistics 1992.* London: HMSO, 1992.
- Department of Social Security. *Notes on the diagnosis of prescribed diseases, 1991.* London: HMSO, 1993.
- Health and Safety Executive. *A guide to the reporting of injuries, diseases and dangerous occurrences regulations 1995–1996.* London: HMSO, 1996.

Doctors can obtain further information and help about occupational diseases from the Employment Medical Advisory Service, which is contactable through local branches of the Health and Safety Executive. The Executive produces many publications for doctors, workers, and employers, and these are available from any HMSO outlet. In addition, there are regional specialty advisors in occupational medicine. They can be contacted through the Faculty of Occupational Medicine of the Royal College of Physicians, Regent's Park, London NW1 4LB (telephone (0171) 487 3414), which also issues publications and advice on training. The Society of Occupational Medicine offers membership to anyone interested in health in the workplace.

2 OCCUPATIONAL HEARING LOSS AND VIBRATION INDUCED DISORDERS

C M Jones

Hearing loss

Incidence of occupational hearing loss

- Department of Social Security estimated that 13 000 workers received benefits in 1992
- It is the third commonest assessed claim (after hand-arm vibration syndrome and tenosynovitis)
- The OPCS Disability Survey (1985–8) estimated that 52 500 people were affected in England and Wales
- The 1990 Labour Force survey estimated that 103 100 people had deafness, tinnitus, or other ear conditions caused by work and a further 18 300 thought that their ear condition had been made worse by work

Causes of deafness

Sensorineural loss
- Congenital deafness (associated with maternal rubella or flu or prenatal medication)
- Familial deafness
- Birth trauma
- Childhood illnesses (such as measles (usually bilateral deafness), mumps (unilateral), encephalitis, meningitis, cerebral abscess, typhus)
- Ototoxic drugs
    - Streptomycin and some other antibiotics (such as gentamicin and neomycin)
    - Anti-rheumatic drugs
    - Diuretics
    - Quinine, nicotine, alcohol, and aspirin
- Fracture of base of skull
- Acoustic neuroma (unilateral deafness)
- Ménière's disease
- Presbycusis

Conductive loss
- Impacted earwax
- Ruptured eardrum (blow to head or explosion)
- Blockage of eustachian tube
- Ossicular dysfunction
    - Dislocation
    - Otitis media or fluid
    - Otosclerosis

Audiometric characteristics of noise induced hearing loss

- Bilateral notch in hearing threshold at 3, 4, or 6 kHz with recovery at 8 kHz
- Progressive deepening and widening of notch with increasing exposure to noise
- Notch due to shooting is narrow and asymmetrical (in right handed people it is deeper on left side because right ear is protected by gun stock)
- The 6 kHz frequency is the most variable tested, and an isolated notch at 6 kHz is usually of no clinical importance

In 1908 the annual report of the Chief Inspector of Factories stated: "men employed in certain trades are liable to have their sense of hearing seriously impaired, if not entirely destroyed in the course of time, as a result of long continued exposure to loud noise." It is only in recent decades that this situation has begun to change.

This irreversible sensorineural deafness is caused by damage to the hair cells of the organ of Corti in the cochlea. It can be the cause of accidents due to failure to hear warning signals. It reduces the quality of life and, especially in elderly people, produces social isolation. If tinnitus is prominent psychiatric symptoms can occur.

Clinical presentation

Noise induced hearing loss develops insidiously. A gradual loss of clarity in perceived speech occurs, which is often attributed to inattention or to others not speaking clearly because when the sufferer looks at speakers he or she can understand them. Difficulty in understanding others in a crowd is, in the same way, presumed to be due to competition with background noise (perceptual rivalry). Eventually, the sufferer realises that others do not have this problem. This realisation may come suddenly, such as when a telephone with an electronic bleep is bought to replace one with a bell.

A high pitched tinnitus, initially intermittent, becomes continuous in up to 20% of cases and can be a presenting symptom. The other feature (usually revealed on direct questioning) is loudness recruitment: at a certain volume perceived sound suddenly becomes more intense.

Diagnosis

As well as asking about current symptoms, the doctor taking a patient's history should cover other possible causes of sensorineural and conductive deafness. Both social and work related exposure to noise should be reviewed, including the firing of guns (military and sporting), playing in pop groups, and listening to amplified music. To help assess the level of noise at work, a useful rule of thumb is that voices need to be raised to communicate over a distance of one metre at 90 dB(A).

A check should be made of the present and past use of hearing protectors, their type, and how often they are used.

Examination by otoscopy and tuning fork tests can exclude other causes of deafness. The diagnosis is usually made by air and bone conduction audiometry being compatible with exposure to noise, although other tests, such as cortical electrical response audiometry, may be advisable in some cases.

Audiometry

Audiometry should be performed when the subject has not been exposed to loud noise for at least 16 hours (or has worn high efficiency muffs before the test). This minimises the temporary lowering of the hearing threshold caused by noise (temporary threshold shift).

There is a learning effect with audiometry. This can result in the thresholds for the second ear tested (conventionally the right ear) being better than the first. The learning effect can also extend to the next two audiometric tests. It may be up to 10–15 dB for each frequency.

Audiometric screening in industry is usually done by discrete frequency, pulsed tone, self recording, air conducting audiometry according to the Bekesey or Hughson-Westlake procedure. Accuracy is related to the background level of noise during testing, and so a soundproof booth is usually required (EN 26189 gives the criteria).

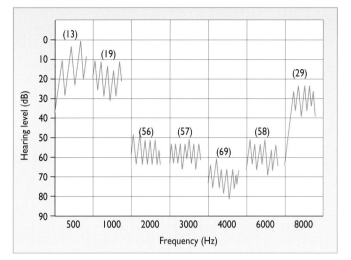

Audiogram of 50 year old man with disability of 44 dB. Pattern is typical of noise induced hearing loss.

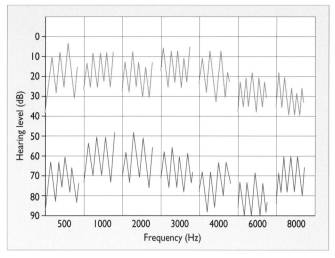

Audiogram showing conductive pattern of hearing loss after acute perforation of eardrum (red) compared with normal pattern for a 54 year old man (blue).

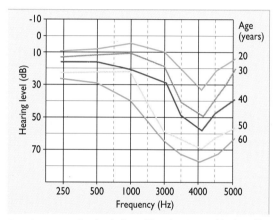

Development of noise induced hearing loss with time (for exposure to 101 dB(A) and including presbycusis).

A loss of less than 20 dB in all frequencies can be considered normal. A similar reduction in all frequencies or one where the threshold improves in the higher frequencies indicates a conductive loss. A notch in the region of 1–3 kHz indicates a familial cause of hearing loss. Classic noise induced hearing loss occurs at 4 kHz. Presbycusis produces a smooth pattern of increasing loss in higher frequencies.

The population varies considerably in its susceptibility to the effect of noise (as shown by the distribution of men's average threshold for 1–3 kHz in the box, bottom left). The rate of hearing loss due to noise is greatest at initial exposure and reduces progressively with continued exposure. In contrast the changes due to presbycusis increase progressively and must always be considered when audiograms are interpreted. The progression is less in women and in people living in rural areas. As presbycusis affects the higher noise frequencies, most of its effect on the calculation of disability can usually be ignored during working life.

Average correction (in dB) for presbycusis

Age (years)	Noise frequency (kHz)						
	0·5	1	2	3	4	6	8
30	1	1	1	2	2	3	3
40	2	2	3	6	8	9	11
50	4	4	7	12	16	18	23
60	6	7	12	20	28	32	39
70	10	11	19	31	43	49	60

Calculation of disability for compensation awarded by Department of Social Security

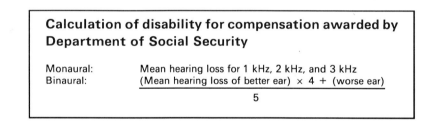

Monaural: Mean hearing loss for 1 kHz, 2 kHz, and 3 kHz

Binaural: $\dfrac{(\text{Mean hearing loss of better ear}) \times 4 + (\text{worse ear})}{5}$

Disability and compensation

Disability is calculated from the hearing loss in the main speech frequencies (1–3 kHz). Tinnitus adds to this. Disability should be calculated only from an audiogram produced after 48 hours without noise exposure (to exclude the temporary threshold shift) and preferably one that is not the first audiogram recorded for the patient (to allow for the learning effect). If the impairment is about the same in both ears and there is no tinnitus, it is unusual for the sufferer to experience significant handicap with less than 20 dB of disability. At 50 dB the handicap is substantial, and lip reading is required for comprehension of speech. The Department of Social Security awards compensation when disability exceeds 50 dB but calculates the size of award from a disability of 30 dB. Many sufferers do not apply for compensation because they know the conditions are stringent.

In recent years, because of the high cost of litigation, most compensation has been provided by agreements between unions and insurance companies, and impairments as low as 10–14 dB have been compensated. However, the trend is now against this because of the increasing value of awards given in the civil courts.

Average hearing threshold (in dB) for 1–3 kHz for men exposed to 90 dB(A)

Age (years)	Population centiles				
	10	30	50	70	90
20	11	6	3	0	−3
30	23	15	10	6	2
40	33	22	16	11	6
50	42	29	22	16	10
60	51	38	30	24	16

Noise in the workplace

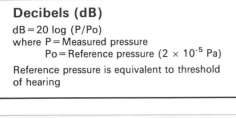

Decibels (dB)

$dB = 20 \log (P/Po)$
where P = Measured pressure
Po = Reference pressure (2×10^{-5} Pa)

Reference pressure is equivalent to threshold of hearing

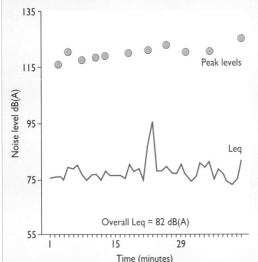

Relation between short term Leqs, period Leq, and peak sound level in an industrial situation.

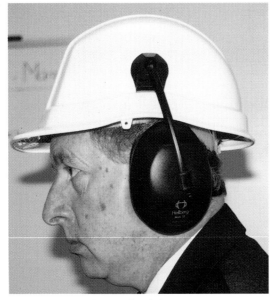

Ear muffs attached to a safety helmet.

1989 Noise at Work Regulations

Employers have a general duty to
• Make, review, and record assessments of noise
• Reduce damage to hearing of employees
• Reduce exposure to noise by methods other than use of ear protectors
• Provide hearing protection
• Create "ear protection zones"
• Use and maintain equipment for reducing exposure to noise
• Provide information, instruction, and training

Manufacturers are required to provide noise levels of equipment that they have supplied

Assessing noise exposure

Because of the ear's range of sensitivity, noise is measured on the logarithmic decibel scale, in which 0 is the limit of detection and about 130–135 dB is painful. As the ear has varying sensitivity to different sound frequencies, weighting factors are applied to each frequency to derive the dB(A) scale, in which all frequencies sound equally loud. An increase of 3 dB(A) is only just detectable to the human ear, though this is equivalent to a doubling of the sound intensity.

Hearing damage is related to the total noise dose received at the ear—a product of the noise level and its duration. Explosive noise is more damaging than continuous noise as the stapedial reflex (which reduces transmission of intense sound) takes 10 milliseconds to activate.

The Leq (the equivalent continuous sound level) is a single value that has the same energy level as the fluctuating levels normally experienced (the time weighted average). It can be calculated over any period of time, but modern sound level meters can measure it directly.

Legislation is formulated on the basis of an Leq for an eight hour day (the $L_{EP,d}$) and the maximum instantaneous (peak) noise level.

Noise in the workplace is assessed with sound level meters of varying complexity. A personal dosimeter may be attached to a person, or tape recordings can be taken for later analysis. A doctor needs to know the $L_{EP,d}$, the peak level, and the frequency distribution of the noise.

Preventing hearing loss

The use of ear protectors should be considered as a last resort when the engineering control of noise is inadequate. In reality, however, ear protectors are commonly needed because fully controlling noise at source can be very difficult and expensive.

Various types of protectors are available. Ear muffs, with oil or foam filled seals, are attached to head bands or helmets. Ear plugs—which may be disposable, reusable, or made to measure—and ear caps attached to stethoscope bands are also available. Manufacturers provide the mean and standard deviation of their ability to attenuate the standard frequencies or a single number rating (NNR). The level of protection is conventionally considered to be the "mean−(1 SD)" per frequency.

The selected ear protector should be appropriate for both the frequency and level of the noise and should attenuate sounds to about 80 dB(A). Any greater attenuation can cause social isolation. There is increasing evidence that some ear plugs are not as effective in practice as test figures suggest, and some companies prohibit their use for high noise levels. Protectors must be worn continuously to be effective: unprotected exposure to 100 dB(A) for 15 minutes is equivalent to eight hours of exposure at 85 dB(A), and even the best protector worn for half of the time will reduce the $L_{EP,d}$ by only 3–5 dB(A).

Legal considerations

Until the 1989 Noise at Work Regulations were introduced after the 1986 European Commission directive, only a voluntary code of practice published by the Department of Employment (1972) and the 1974 Woodworking Regulations applied.

The current regulations state that
• At the first action level ($L_{EP,d}$ of 85 dB(A)) an assessment should be made by a competent person, advice be given to employees, ear protectors be made available, and noise reduction be effected if reasonably practicable
• At the second action level ($L_{EP;d}$ of 90 dB(A)) the full requirements of the legislation are invoked (see box), and ear protection must be worn
• If the peak sound pressure exceeds 200 pascals (that is, 140 dB relative to 20 µPa) the full requirements apply regardless of the $L_{EP,d}$.

Many employers implement a comprehensive hearing conservation programme with routine audiometry.

Hand-arm vibration syndrome

Classification of hand-arm vibration syndrome (Stockholm scale)

Vascular component

Stage (grade)	Description
0	No attacks
1V (mild)	Occasional attacks affecting only tips of one or more fingers
2V (moderate)	Occasional attacks affecting distal and middle (rarely also proximal) phalanges of one or more fingers
3V (severe)	Frequent attacks affecting all phalanges of most fingers
4V (very severe)	As in stage 3 but with trophic changes in fingertips

Sensorineural component

Stage	Description
OSN	Exposed to vibration but no symptoms
1SN	Intermittent numbness with or without tingling
2SN	Intermittent or persistent numbness, reduced sensory perception
3SN	Intermittent or persistent numbness, reduced tactile discrimination or manual dexterity

Staging is made separately for each hand. Grade of disorder is indicated by stage and number of affected fingers on both hands.

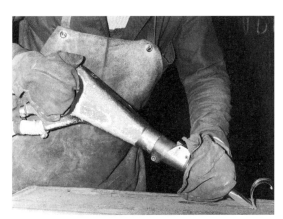

Using a chipping hammer with overhand grip

Differential diagnosis of hand-arm vibration syndrome (most are rare)

Vascular
- Trauma
- Polyarteritis nodosa
- Scleroderma
- Thoracic outlet syndrome
- Cold agglutinins
- Systemic lupus erythematosus
- Dermatomyositis
- Rheumatoid arthritis

Neurological
- Peripheral nerve entrapment
- Trauma to arm or neck
- Peripheral neuropathy
- Drugs and other toxic effects
- Syringomyelia
- Spinal cord compression
- Multiple sclerosis

Further reading
- *The noise at work regulations.* London: HMSO, 1990. (Noise guides Nos 1–8)
- *Management of health and safety at work regulations and approved code of practice.* London: HMSO, 1992.
- *Hand transmitted vibration clinical effects and pathophysiology.* Parts 1 and 2. London: Faculty of Occupational Medicine Royal College of Physicians of London, 1993.

Until recently this was known as vibration induced white finger (VIWF), reflecting its mode of presentation. It has been renamed to reflect the wider range of its effects. The Taylor-Pelmear classification is also being replaced by the Stockholm Workshop scale.

Though originally described in the mining, metallurgical, and engineering industries, forestry may now be the main source of cases because of widespread use of chainsaws. How vibration actually induces the condition is not clear, but recent studies suggest it is probably a local effect on nerves and blood vessels.

Presentation

The presentation is of progressive Raynaud's phenomenon in an operator of vibrating tools. After a latent period, vasospasm is first noticed on cold, wet, and windy mornings in the tips of the fingers most affected by vibration. Intermittent numbness or tingling often precedes actual blanching.

With continued exposure to vibration, the vasospasm progresses proximally and to other fingers, but the thumb is rarely affected. The vasospasm is rarely symmetrical and has a characteristic pattern that reflects the subject's grip on the vibrating tool—thus, an underhand grip on a vibrating chisel affects mainly the index finger, whereas the little finger is mainly affected with an overhand grip. After the painless vasospasm ("dead finger"), a cyanotic phase may occur before a painful hyperaemia ("hot aches"). In some cases only cyanosis occurs with vasospasm. In the most severe cases the fingers are permanently cyanosed and trophic changes of the fingertips can occur. The intermittent neuropathy that accompanies the vasospasm becomes continuous and deteriorates with further exposure. It affects most modalities and results in clumsiness.

Unless it is associated with cold, vibration itself rarely induces vasospasm. As the condition develops, the amount of cold required to induce vasospasm is less and the condition can occur in the summer, though usually in association with wet hands or wind.

Diagnosis

This is usually made by the history being characteristic and compatible with the exposure to vibration and excluding other causes. There is no single clinical diagnostic test. Carpal tunnel syndrome, itself reportable under RIDDOR for vibration exposed workers, should be excluded.

Prognosis

The vascular component can slowly improve if exposure to vibration is stopped early in stage 2, and a change of job should be encouraged. It is debatable whether the neurological symptoms can improve.

Assessing risk

Risk of the condition is related to the vibration dose received by the hand, the strength of grip used, the type of vibration, the ratio of work and rest periods, and factors affecting the circulation such as body warmth and smoking. There is great individual variation. The condition seems to be more common with low frequency vibrations but has been reported with frequencies up to 1500 Hz. Accelerometer readings can be taken on a vibrating tool or the interface between hand and tool to evaluate the potential risk.

3 OCCUPATIONAL ASTHMA AND OTHER RESPIRATORY DISEASES

Ira Madan

Changing pattern of occupational lung disease

Cases of work related respiratory disease in United Kingdom in 1994 (based on Ross et al[1])	
Disease	Estimated No of cases
Occupational asthma	941
Non-malignant pleural disease	730
Mesothelioma	644
Pneumoconiosis	341
Inhalation accidents	280
Other diagnosis	109
Lung cancer	70
Infectious disease	59
Extrinsic allergic alveolitis	46
Bronchitis	38
Building related illness	8
Byssinosis	1
Total	3267

In the United Kingdom, over the past 40 years, there has been a shift away from manufacturing industries and a sharp reduction in the numbers of coal miners. These factors, together with stricter health and safety legislation, have resulted in a substantial decline in the prevalence of silicosis and pneumoconiosis. In contrast, occupational asthma has become increasingly recognised. In developing countries, however, the traditional occupational lung diseases of silicosis, pneumoconiosis, and asbestosis remain common in rapidly industrialising areas.

Our understanding of the epidemiology of occupational lung disease in Britain has been greatly enhanced by the SWORD project (surveillance of work related and occupational respiratory disease), which was established in 1989 sponsored by the Health and Safety Executive. Occupational and respiratory physicians are invited to report new cases of occupational lung diseases together with the suspected agent. The data are regularly analysed and the results published. Further information is available from the Department of Occupational and Environmental Medicine, National Heart and Lung Institute, London.

Occupational asthma

Major causes of occupational asthma and groups at risk in 1993-4 (based on Sallie et al[2])		
Causative agent	Main occupations	
Isocyanates	Coach and other paint spraying	18%
Laboratory animals	Laboratory technicians and assistants	9%
Grain	Baking and milling	9%
Hardening agents, glues, and resins	Manufacturing and processing plastics	8%
Wood dust	Joinery	5%
Soldering flux	Welding, soldering, electronic assembly	4%
Glutaraldehyde	Nursing	3%
Enzymes	Miscellaneous	2%

Occupational asthma is caused by specific sensitising agents inhaled in the workplace—it does not include bronchoconstriction induced by irritants such as exercise and cold air that are encountered at work. There are over 200 known respiratory sensitisers, and more are identified each year. Some sensitisers may not be immediately obvious: thus, it has recently been recognised that workers such as those in health services can develop occupational asthma as a result of wearing latex gloves. The allergen is latex protein, which becomes airborne as the gloves are used.

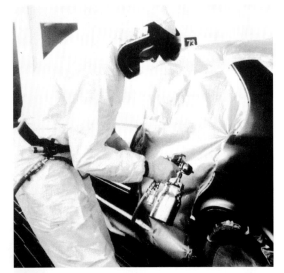
Worker properly protected from di-isocyanates in spray paint.

Diagnosis

A comprehensive and detailed occupational history is essential in the initial assessment of a worker thought to have occupational asthma. Coughing at work or at the end of a shift is often the first symptom and precedes wheezing. Concurrent rhinorrhoea, nasal congestion, and lacrimation may be associated with exposure to substances of high molecular weight—such as rat urinary proteins. The symptoms generally improve at weekends and holidays, but at advanced stages the respiratory symptoms may persist. Physical examination is rarely helpful—even in confirmed cases the chest often seems to be normal.

All aspects of a patient's job, including processes in adjacent areas, should be reviewed to identify tasks that could lead to exposure to a sensitising agent. Information about previous jobs should be obtained to determine whether there has been prior exposure to such agents. If a company employs an occupational health service, advice should be sought from the occupational physician, who will have information on the substances that employees are exposed to, including COSHH (control of substances hazardous to health) assessments. The physician may also know whether any other workers have developed occupational asthma.

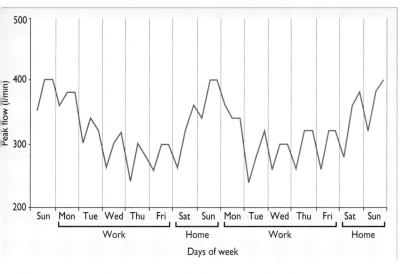

Self recorded peak flow measurements showing classic pattern of occupational asthma.

Investigations

Patients should record the best of three measurements of peak expiratory flow made every two to three hours from waking to sleeping over a period of one month. Ideally, this period should include one or two weeks away from work. A drop in peak expiratory flow or substantial diurnal variability in peak expiratory flow on working days but not on days away from work supports a diagnosis of occupational asthma. The times of working shifts and use of any drugs must be considered when the records of peak expiratory flow are reviewed.

If there is any doubt about the diagnosis and the patient's company does not have access to an occupational physician, the patient should be referred to a consultant occupational physician or respiratory physician. Further specialist investigations include immunological testing and, if the diagnosis is uncertain, bronchial challenge with the suspected agent.

A worker who develops occupational asthma should avoid further exposure to the causative agent. As this often means relocation or loss of current employment, it is essential that the specific cause is accurately identified

---

Management

Although treatment of acute occupational asthma is the same as for asthma generally, it is important to be aware that, once a person has been sensitised to a specific substance, subsequent exposure to even minimal quantities of the substance may precipitate severe bronchoconstriction. A company's occupational physician will be able to advise on suitable areas for redeployment and may be able to arrange this with the employee's manager.

Occupational asthma is a prescribed occupational disease. A worker who develops the condition is entitled to "no fault" compensation if the degree of disability is considered to be 14% or over.

Pneumoconiosis

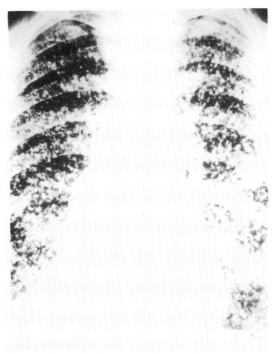

Chest radiograph of quarry worker showing extensive simple silicosis.

Pneumoconiosis is the generic term for the lodgement of any inhaled dusts in the lungs irrespective of the effects (excluding asthma and neoplasia). Sporadic cases of chronic silicosis (fibrosis of the lungs due to inhalation of silicon dioxide) still occur in Britain, usually in people working with slate or granite and in fettlers in foundries. Patients present with increasing dyspnoea over several years, and chest radiographs reveal upper lobe fibrosis or calcified nodules.

The chronic pneumoconiosis of coal miners, due to inhalation of coal dust, produces no symptoms or physical signs: its only danger is that it predisposes to progressive massive fibrosis, which, when sufficiently advanced, causes dyspnoea and cor pulmonale. However, this condition is disappearing in Britain as mines are closed.

Acute silicosis results from a brief but heavy exposure, such as occurs in sandblasting without respiratory protection. Such patients become intensely breathless and may die within months. Chest radiographs show an appearance like pulmonary oedema. As with many other occupational lung diseases, several recent episodes of silicosis could have been avoided if employers had provided satisfactory ventilation in the workplace.

Extrinsic allergic alveolitis

Extrinsic allergic alveolitis is a granulomatous inflammatory reaction caused by an immunological response to inhaled organic dusts or chemicals. Farmer's lung and bird fancier's lung remain the most prevalent forms of the disease. The condition should be suspected if flu-like symptoms occur after exposure to microbial spores, animal proteins, or certain chemicals. Prolonged illness may be associated with considerable weight loss, but symptoms usually tend to improve within 48 hours of removal from the causative agent.

Inspiratory crackles may be heard on examination of the chest, and a chest radiograph may show a ground glass pattern or micronodular shadows. The diagnosis is confirmed by a reduction in lung volumes, impairment of gas transfer, and demonstration of precipitating antibodies (precipitins) to the causal agent in the serum.

Common causes of extrinsic allergic alveolitis

Disease	Source of antigen	Antigen
Farmer's lung	Mouldy hay and straw	*Micropolyspora faeni Thermoactinomyces vulgaris*
Bird fancier's lung	Bird excreta and bloom	Bird serum proteins
Mushrooms worker's lung	Spores released during spawning	Thermophilic actinomycetes
Ventilation pneumonitis	Contaminated air conditioning systems	Thermophilic actinomycetes

Effects of asbestos

Occupational groups at greatest risk of developing asbestos related diseases

- Carpenters and electricians
- Builders
- Gas fitters
- Roofers
- Demolition workers
- Shipyard and rail workers
- Insulation workers
- Asbestos factory workers

Any patient with a history of exposure to asbestos should be encouraged to stop smoking as these two factors have a synergistic effect in development of lung cancer

Non-malignant disorders

Non-malignant asbestos related disorders consist of asbestosis, pleural plaques, diffuse thickening of the pleura, benign pleural effusions, and asbestos corns (callosities on the dorsal and palmar surfaces of the hands, which may be tender to pressure).

Asbestosis is a diffuse interstitial pulmonary fibrosis caused by exposure to fibres of asbestos, and its diagnosis is helped by obtaining a history of regular exposure to any form of airborne asbestos. The presence of calcified pleural plaques on a chest radiograph indicates exposure to asbestos and may help to distinguish the condition from other causes of pulmonary fibrosis.

Malignant disorders

The malignant asbestos related disorders are bronchial cancer and malignant mesothelioma of the pleura and peritoneum. It is essential to obtain a full occupational history from any patient with a diagnosis of primary lung cancer: if there is evidence of asbestosis or bilateral diffuse pleural thickening and a history of exposure to asbestos at work, the patient may be eligible for compensation from the Department of Social Security. This also applies to patients with primary lung cancer who have evidence of silicosis and who have been exposed to silica dust at work.

Mesothelioma

Most cases of mesothelioma are pleural in origin, and the disease usually develops 20-40 years after exposure to perhaps even small amounts of blue (crocidolite) or brown (amosite) asbestos. The incidence of the disease is still increasing in men born before 1948, and recent research has indicated that deaths from mesothelioma will increase for at least another 15-25 years.

The disease is often insidious—breathlessness and chest pain are the commonest symptoms, and patients usually have a pleural effusion by the time they present to their general practitioner. The diagnosis is made by a history of exposure to asbestos, the clinical picture described, and radiography (including, if necessary, computed tomography).

Treatment is largely palliative as most people die within a year of diagnosis. All cases of mesothelioma in Britain are assumed to be due to occupation, and patients are eligible for industrial injuries benefit from the Department of Social Security provided that the diagnosis is reasonably certain and there is a history of appropriate exposure.

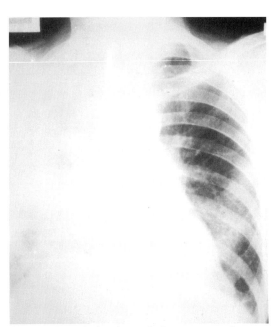

Chest radiograph showing typical appearance of mesothelioma

Exposure to gases

> Inhalation or irritant gases such as chlorine may result in pulmonary oedema

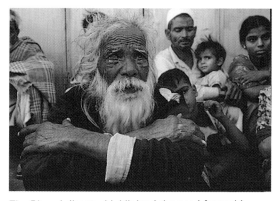

The Bhopal disaster highlighted the need for rapid access to expert advice in the event of a chemical disaster.

Although fatalities from exposure to gases in the workplace are now rare in Britain, inhalation accidents still occur relatively frequently. Asthma may develop within hours of inhaling a toxic chemical in a high concentration. The resulting airway hyperresponsiveness, known as reactive airways dysfunction syndrome, usually resolves spontaneously but can persist indefinitely.

On a wider scale, industrial accidents involving the release of a toxic irritant gas may cause pulmonary injury or even death in the surrounding population. One of the worst recent examples was the release of methyl isocyanate from the Union Carbide pesticide plant in Bhopal, India, in 1984. Many victims died of acute pulmonary oedema. Survivors suffered from chronic respiratory ill health with chest pain, haemoptysis, and, in the longer term, bronchiolitis obliterans.

Key references

1 Ross DJ, Sallie BA, McDonald JC. SWORD'94: surveillance of work-related and occupational respiratory disease in the UK. Occup Med 1995; 45:175–8.
2 Sallie BA, Ross DJ, Meredith SK, McDonald JC. SWORD'93: surveillance of work-related and occupational respiratory disease in the UK. Occup Med 1994;44:177–82.

The picture of victims of the Bhopal disaster is reproduced with permission of Rex Features.

4 BACK PAIN

Malcolm I V Jayson

Epidemiology of back disability

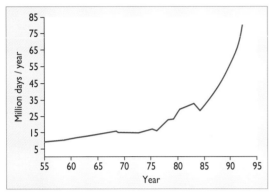

Changes in sickness and invalidity benefit for back pain since 1955 (from report of Clinical Standards Advisory Group[1]).

The number of working days lost due to back problems has increased dramatically in recent years. Over 80 million days a year are now lost due to registered disability,[1] but the total estimate, including short spells, is probably in the order of 150 million. This is some four times the figure for 20 years ago. This increase does not reflect an increased incidence of back problems, which has changed little over the period, but rather increased disability associated with episodes of back pain. Much of the increase in disability is probably due to an altered reaction to the problem, with increases in sick certification and state benefit perhaps reflecting patients' and doctors' expectations, concerns by employers, and social and medicolegal pressures.

The costs of back pain are huge. Current estimates suggest the global cost to our economy is about £6bn a year.[1] Improved management and better outcomes would lead to major financial, as well as medical, benefits.

Who gets back pain?

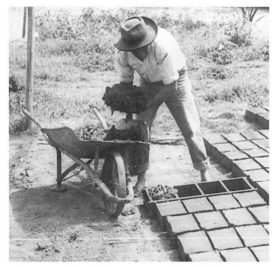

Heavy manual work increases people's risk of back disability.

The problem affects workers of all ages. It usually starts between the late teens and the 40s, with the peak prevalence in 45-60 year olds and little difference between the sexes. There is an increased prevalence of back disability in people performing heavy manual work, smokers, and those in social classes IV and V. Clearly, these factors interact in many patients. It is often difficult to determine whether heavy manual work has caused or aggravated a back problem or whether a worker cannot do the job because of back pain. Obesity and tallness are also associated with back problems. Postural abnormalities, however, do not predict back problems, except possibly gross discrepancies in leg length.

Psychological factors are important. Psychological distress in a population without back pain predicts the development of back pain.[2] In the Boeing aircraft factory, workers who did not enjoy their jobs had a greatly increased risk of reporting back injury.[3]

Causes of back pain

The major causes of back pain are mechanical strains and sprains, lumbar spondylosis, herniated intervertebral disc, and spinal stenosis. In many cases it is not possible to make a specific mechanical diagnosis. Such problems are commonly called non-specific back pain. Non-mechanical causes of back pain include inflammatory disorders such as ankylosing spondylitis and infections, primary and secondary neoplasms, and metabolic bone disorders such as osteoporosis. The patient's clinical characteristics and a general health screen will exclude systemic disease.

Pre-employment screening

There is no evidence that physical build, flexibility of spine movements, or other physical characteristics are of any value in predicting the development of back problems, and they should not be used for screening purposes. In particular, lumbar radiographs are not helpful in identifying people liable to develop back pain at work.

All subjects should have a detailed medical and occupational history taken and should be assessed as to whether they are fit enough to do the job. The most useful single item of information in predicting potential back problems is a history of back pain, particularly if it was recent and severe enough to cause absence from work.[4]

> The physical state of the spine determines how well it functions, and use and injury of the back will alter its structure, This interrelation between structure and function is central to understanding many back problems related to work

> The principal risk factor for back pain is a past history of back pain. Those who have suffered back problems in the past are likely to experience further episodes in the future

Preventing back injuries

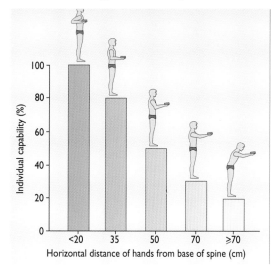

Reduction in handling capacity as hands move away from trunk (from *Manual Handling. Guidance on Regulations*[5]).

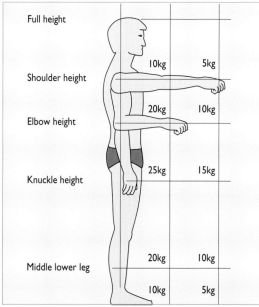

Guide to loads that may be lifted in various positions, assuming that load is easily grasped with both hands (from *Manual Handling. Guidance on Regulations*[5]).

Manual handling is commonly associated with strains and sprains of the back and resultant disability. *Manual Handling. Guidance on Regulations* lists measures that employers should take to reduce the risk of problems.[5] These include
● Avoiding hazardous manual handling operations as far as is reasonably possible—lifting aids may be appropriate
● Making an appropriate assessment of any hazardous manual handling operations that cannot be avoided
● Reducing the risks of injuries from these operations as far as is reasonably possible.

Weight limits

In Britain there are no specified limits for weights that may be lifted. This is because setting a weight limit is a fallacious approach as so much depends on the individual and the circumstances of any procedure. When a load is moved away from the trunk the level of stress on the lower back increases. As a rough guide, holding a load at arms' length imposes five times the stress experienced with the same load held close to the trunk. Moreover, the further away the load is from the trunk the less easy it is to control, adding to the problems.

Guidelines to loads that may be lifted are necessarily crude given the wide range of individual physical capabilities even among fit and healthy people. There are no truly safe loads, but the stated thresholds provide reasonable protection to nearly all men and between a half and two thirds of women. However, many episodes of pain arise in relation to lesser movements, and in these cases it is likely that the spine was vulnerable and at risk of developing problems.

Lifting technique

The technique of lifting is important. Simple ergonomic principles will protect the back against excessive stresses. A poor posture increases the risk of injury. Examples include stooping and twisting while weight bearing, carrying loads in an asymmetric fashion, moving loads excessive distances, and excessive pushing and pulling. Repeated or prolonged physical effort may carry additional risk. Many episodes of back pain develop after sudden or unanticipated movements such as a stumble on the stairs or an unexpected twist.

Wherever manual handling occurs employers should consider the risks of injury and how to reduce them by reviewing the task required, the load carried, the working environment, and individual capability. Redesigning the job and providing mechanical assistance may be appropriate, and individual workers should be trained in safe manual handling.

Place the feet. Feet apart, giving a balanced and stable base for lifting, leading leg as far forward as is comfortable.

Adopt a good posture. Bend the knees so that the hands when grasping the load are as nearly level with the waist as possible. Do not kneel or overflex the knees. Keep the back straight. Lean forward a little over the load if necessary to get a good grip. Keep shoulders level and facing in the same direction as the hips.

Get a firm grip. Try to keep the arms within the boundary formed by the legs. The optimum grip depends on the circumstances, but it must be secure. A hook grip is less fatiguing than keeping the fingers straight. If it is necessary to vary the grip as the lift proceeds, do this as smoothly as possible.

Don't jerk. Carry out the lifting movement smoothly, keeping control of the load.

Move the feet. Don't twist the trunk when turning to the side.

Keep close to the load. Keep the load close to the trunk for as long as possible. Keep the heaviest side of the load next to the trunk. If a close approach to the load is not possible try sliding it towards you before attempting to lift it.

Principles of lifting and carrying a load (adapted from *Manual Handling. Guidance on Regulations*[5]).

Diagnosis and prognosis

Characteristics of simple backache

- Onset generally at ages 20-55
- Pain in lumbosacral region, buttocks, and thighs
- Pain is mechanical in nature—varies with physical activity and with time
- Patient is well
- Prognosis is good—90% of patients recover from acute attack in six weeks

---

Characteristics of nerve root pain

- Unilateral leg pain worse than back pain
- Pain generally radiates to foot or toes
- Numbness and paraesthesia in same distribution
- Signs of nerve irritation—reduced straight leg raise which reproduces leg pain
- Motor, sensory, or reflex change—limited to one nerve foot
- Prognosis reasonable—50% of patients recover from acute attack in six weeks

---

Red flags suggesting possible serious spinal pathology

- Age at onset <20 or >55
- Violent trauma—such as fall from height or road traffic accident
- Constant, progressive, non-mechanical pain
- Thoracic pain
- Past history of cancer
- Use of systemic corticosteroids
- Misuse of drugs, infection with HIV
- Patient systematically unwell
- Weight loss
- Persisting severe restriction of lumbar flexion
- Widespread neurological signs
- Structural deformity

Management

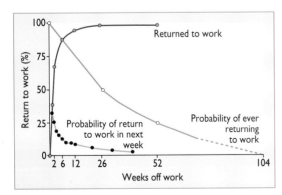
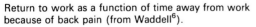

Return to work as a function of time away from work because of back pain (from Waddell[6]).

Diagnostic triage

On simple clinical grounds patients with acute back problems can be triaged into simple backache, nerve root pain, and possible serious spinal pathology. Simple backache will be managed by an occupational physician or general practitioner. Nerve root pain will initially be dealt with by a general practitioner in a similar way to simple backache, though at a slower pace, providing there is no major or progressive motor weakness. However, early referral to a specialist may be required. Urgent referrals are necessary for patients with possible serious spinal pathology, and emergency referral is needed for those with widespread or progressive neurological changes.

Indications for emergency referral

- Difficulty with micturition
- Loss of anal sphincter tone or faecal incontinence
- Saddle anaesthesia about anus, perineum, or genitals
- Widespread (more than one nerve root) or progressive motor weakness in legs or disturbed gait

---

Prognosis

Most patients have simple backache. The exact pathology and the exact source of the pain are rarely identifiable, but the principles of management are now well established. Nearly all episodes of acute back pain resolve rapidly. Most patients return to work within a few days, and 90% return within six weeks. Some patients, however, develop chronic back pain, and this small proportion with prolonged disability are responsible for most of the costs associated with back injuries.

With longer time off work, the chances of ever getting back to work decrease rapidly. Only 25% of those off work for a year and 10% of those off work for two years will return to productive employment.[1]

Investigations

Routine *x* ray investigations of the lumbar spine should be avoided. Apparent degenerative changes are common and correlate poorly with symptoms—they are better considered as age related changes. Radiographs are necessary when there is the question of possible serious spinal pathology, but a negative result does not exclude infection or tumour.

Imaging with computed tomography or magnetic resonance imaging is of no value for simple backache. These techniques also often show age related changes that correlate poorly with symptoms. The presence of these changes does not influence management.

Simple backache

The early management of acute back pain is all important. Much of the traditional management of back pain seems to promote chronicity. In view of the increasing toll of back disability, the Clinical Standards Advisory Group of the Department of Health has published guidelines on managing back problems.[1] These emphasise the importance of maintaining physical activity and minimising the period off work.

The natural course of simple backache is spontaneous resolution within a short time. Treatment is directed at relief of symptoms, a minimum period of rest, physical activity, and rapid return to work.

Pain relief is with simple analgesics such as paracetamol or possibly with non-steroidal anti-inflammatory drugs. Avoid narcotics if possible, and never use them for more than two weeks.

Rest is prescribed only if essential. Bed rest should be limited to one to three days as longer periods increase the duration of disability.[7]

Early activity is encouraged. Patients should be reassured that exercise promotes recovery. The particular type of exercise is less important. There may be some increase in pain, but patients should be reassured that hurt does not mean harm and that those who exercise have fewer recurrences, take less time off work, and require less health care in the future.

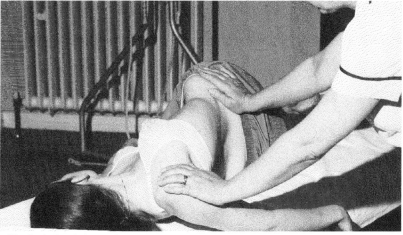

Manipulation helps patients with back disability to mobilise more quickly.

Physical therapy should be arranged if symptoms last for more than a few days. This may include manipulation, exercises, and encouraging physical activity. Other techniques—such as short wave diathermy, infrared, ice packs, ultrasound, massage, and traction provide only transient symptomatic benefit but may enable patients to exercise and mobilise more rapidly. Some factories employ therapists so that physical therapy is available early in the work environment. This approach seems promising in promoting quick recovery and reducing the risks of chronicity.

Risk factors for back pain becoming chronic

- Prior history of low back pain
- Previous time off work because of back pain
- Radicular pain, possibly with reduced straight leg raise and neurological signs
- Poor physical fitness
- Poor general health
- Smoking
- Psychological distress and depression
- Disproportionate pain behaviour
- Low job satisfaction
- Personal problems–alcohol intake, marital, financial
- Medicolegal proceedings

Key references

1 Clinical Standards Advisory Group. *Back pain.* London: HMSO, 1994.
2 Croft PR, Papageorgiou AC, Ferry S, Thomas E, Jayson MIV, Silman A. Psychological distress and low back pain: evidence from a prospective study in general practice. *Spine* 1996;**20**: 2731–7
3 Bigos SJ, Battie MC, Spengler D, Fisher LD, Fordyce WE, Hansson TH, *et al.* A prospective study of work perceptions and psycho-social factors affecting the report of back injury. *Spine* 1991; **16**:1–6
4 Heliovaara M, Makela M, Kenkt P, Impivaara O, Aromaa A. Determinants of sciatica and back pain. *Spine* 1991; **16**: 608–14.
5 Health and Safety Executive. *Manual handling. Guidance on regulations.* London: HMSO, 1992.
6 Waddell G. 1987 Volvo award in clinical sciences. A new clinical model for the treatment of low-back pain. *Spine* 1987;**12**:632–44.
7 Deyo RA, Diehl AJ, Rosenthal M. How many days of bed rest for acute low back pain? *N Engl J Med* 1986;**315**:1064–70.

Persistent back pain

By six weeks, most patients will have recovered and be back at work. A detailed review is required for those with persistent problems. These patients should undergo a bio-psycho-social assessment. There are particular risk factors for chronicity of back pain and more prolonged disability, and their early identification will help in planning treatment.

Biological assessment includes reviewing the diagnostic triage, seeking evidence of nerve root problems or possible serious spinal pathology with appropriate referral. At this stage, measuring the erythrocyte sedimentation rate and plain x ray pictures are indicated.

Psychological assessment should include patients' attitudes and beliefs about pain. Many patients will not attempt to regain mobility because of unjustified fears about the risks of activity and work. Patients may have psychological distress and depressive symptoms and develop characteristics of abnormal illness behaviour.

Social assessment includes patients' relationships with their families, who may reinforce the patients' disability, and work problems related to the physical demands of the job, job satisfaction, compensation, and medicolegal issues.

Referral

When a patient with simple backache does not return to work within three months, specialist referral is required to provide a second opinion about the diagnosis, to arrange investigations, and to advise on management, reassurance, multidisciplinary rehabilitation, and pain management. If pain in the back is referred to the buttocks or thighs the appropriate specialty is rheumatology, pain management, or rehabilitation medicine. For nerve root pain, the patient should be referred to orthopaedics or neurosurgery.

Psychological and social factors are increasingly recognised as important, and a multidisciplinary rehabilitation programme is likely to be effective. This may include incremental exercise and physical reconditioning, behavioural medicine, and encouragement to return to work.

Work modification

Early return to work should be a priority since the physical and psychological consequences of inactivity and unemployment contribute to further dysfunction. Although patients should be encouraged to exercise, some are not capable of undertaking heavy manual work. Careful ergonomic assessment is necessary to avoid excessive stresses on the back. In particular, care should be taken to minimise tasks that require bending, lifting, and twisting. Light work such as reception or inspection duties—which require sitting, standing, and walking but avoid long periods in any one position—may be appropriate. At this point a coordinated approach with the occupational health department is likely to be very helpful.

5 NECK AND ARM DISORDERS

Mats Hagberg

Terms and definitions

Characteristics of non-specific musculoskeletal pain in neck and shoulder

History
- Pain and stiffness gradually increase during work and are worst at end of working day and week
- Pain localised to cervical spine and angle between neck and shoulder
- Usually no radiation of pain
- Symptoms improved by heat and worsened by cold draughts

Signs
- Tenderness over neck and shoulder muscles
- Reduced range of active movement of cervical spine (normal passive movement)
- No neurological deficits

Diferential diagnosis
- Thoracic outlet syndrome and other nerve entrapments
- Systemic diseases

Specific risk factors

Risk factors for work related neck and arm disorders
- Posture
- Repetitive motion
- Handling loads
- Psychological and social factors
- Task invariability
- Individual susceptibility

Over recent years the use of terms such as repetitive strain injury (RSI) and cumulative trauma disorder have been strongly criticised. Sometimes the terms have even been used synonymously with disease terms such as carpal tunnel syndrome (compression of the median nerve at the wrist) and de Quervain's disease (inflammation of the tendons to the long thumb abductor and the short thumb extensor at the wrist). Neither carpal tunnel syndrome nor de Quervain's disease is necessarily related to repetitive strain or cumulative trauma.

Use of these terms to describe work related musculoskeletal disorders has been criticised because they suggest a pathological mechanism that is usually not proved. A work related musculoskeletal disorder may be caused by a single strain or trauma, not necessarily a repetitive or cumulative one. Furthermore, both psychological and social factors play an important role in the genesis and perpetuation of work related musculoskeletal disorders.

The World Health Organisation considers the cause of work related musculoskeletal diseases to be multifactorial. The work environment and the work performed are important but are not the only factors to be considered. The preferred term for conditions that may be subjectively or objectively influenced or caused by work is work related musculoskeletal disorder. This umbrella term neither defines the pathological mechanism nor the diagnostic criteria.

Certain occupations are associated with a high risk for neck and arm pain. Some risk factors can be identified, but the interaction between different risk factors is not understood and there is not enough data yet to set accurate exposure limits for disease effects.

It is important to recognise that personal characteristics and other environmental and sociocultural factors usually play a role in these disorders. A patient with neck pain may be exposed to an awkward posture at work but also to social stress at home—both factors contribute to sustained contraction of the trapezius muscle, inducing pain and stiffness. The cause of a work related disorder can sometimes be attributed to a specific exposure in a job, but there is often simultaneous exposure to several different factors. Individual factors must also be considered when assessing the history of a patient with a work related disorder and when redesigning a job before such a patient returns to work.

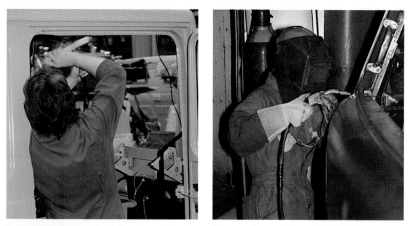

Posture

Working with the hands at or above shoulder level may be one determinant of rotator cuff tendinitis. Industrial workers exposed to tasks that require working over shoulder level include shipyard welders, car assemblers, and house painters. In one study the prevalence of rotator cuff tendinitis was 18% among shipyard welders compared with 2% among male office workers, corresponding to an odds ratio of 13.

Truck assembly and welding – two jobs that often require working with the hands above shoulder height and that are associated with shoulder tendinitis.

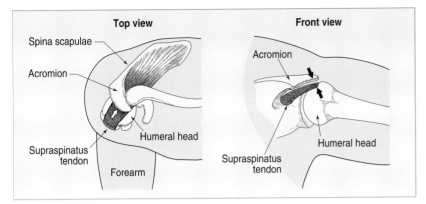

Impingement of supraspinatus tendon against surface of anterior part of acromion when arm is raised to shoulder height. Pressure and mechanical friction are centred on tendon (black arrows).

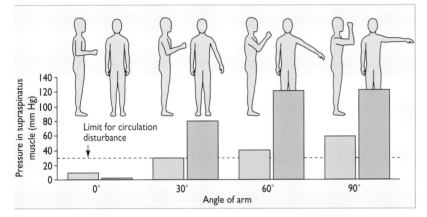

Intramuscular pressure in supraspinatus muscle at different angles of abduction and forward flexion.

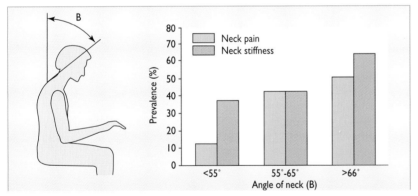

Association between neck flexion and pain and stiffness in neck.

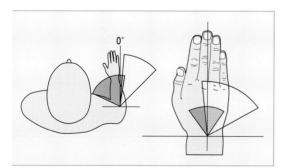

Outward rotation of shoulder and ulnar deviation of wrist found with use of computer mouse (yellow) and keyboard (blue).

The pathogenesis of rotator cuff tendinitis is mainly impingement—the compression of the rotator cuff tendons when they are forced under the coracoacromial arch during elevation of the arm. The supraspinatus tendon is forced under the anterior edge of the acromion, causing both a compression that impairs blood circulation through the tendon and a mechanical friction to the tendon. Reduced blood flow to the tendons because of static muscle contraction may contribute to degeneration of the rotator cuff tendons.

Abduction and forward flexion of more than 30° may constitute a risk factor since the pressure within the supraspinatus muscle will be greater than 30 mmHg, impairing blood flow. The vessels to the supraspinatus tendon run through the muscle, and so the pressure in the muscle can affect tendon vasculature.

Among players of musical instruments, unnatural and constrained postures are common. Pain in the neck and arm have been related to gripping an instrument and awkward posture. Pain in the left shoulder and arm in professional violinists can be due to static holding of the violin in the left hand.

Neck flexion while working at a visual display terminal may be associated with non-specific neck and shoulder symptoms. An exposure-response relation has been found for neck pain and angle of neck flexion among keyboard operators—neck pain was more prevalent among operators who flexed their necks more acutely. Incorrect glasses or need for glasses when working at a visual display terminal may result in neck and shoulder pain.

The development of non-keyboard input devices, such as the computer mouse, has resulted in new postures that may cause a combination of symptoms of the wrist and shoulder. Work tasks of long duration with flexed and, to some extent, extended wrists have been reported as risk factors for carpal tunnel syndrome.

Motion

Repetitive motions of the shoulder may constitute a risk for rotator cuff tendinitis. An experimental study showed that women performing repetitive forward flexions of the shoulder developed shoulder tendinitis. Clinical signs of tendinitis were present up to two weeks after the experiments. Repetitive motions by industrial assembly workers (truck making, meat packing, and circuit board assembly) have been associated with the development of shoulder tendinitis, lateral epicondylitis, and tendinitis at the wrist (de Quervain's disease).

Repetitive motion being a causal factor for tendinitis is consistent with the high risk of shoulder tendinitis among competitive swimmers and epicondylitis among tennis players.

Handling loads

Only a few studies have investigated the effect of handling loads on symptoms of the neck and arms. Handling heavy loads seems to be related to osteoarthrosis and cervical spondylosis. A high risk of acromioclavicular osteoarthrosis and shoulder tendinitis among rock drillers has been attributed to both handling loads and exposure to hand and arm vibration.

Work related musculoskeletal disorders found in blue collar and white collar workers

	Assembly line worker	Keyboard operator
Shoulder pain	Usually shoulder tendinitis due to working with hands above shoulder height	Usually myofascial pain, which may be caused by task invariability leading to static tension of trapezius muscle
Hand and wrist pain	Repetitive power grips may cause repetitive strain of extensor tendons and tendinitis	Intensive keying may cause repetitive strain of extensor tendons and tendinitis
	Carpal tunnel syndrome may also be related to repetitive power grips	Carpal tunnel syndrome may also be related to intensive keying

Psychological and social factors

Psychological and social factors are generally more strongly associated with back pain than shoulder pain. Furthermore, the association is stronger for non-specific pain than for pain with a specific diagnosis. This means that a diagnosis of general cervicobrachial pain may be more strongly related to psychological and social factors than carpal tunnel syndrome or shoulder tendinitis. Highly demanding work and poor work content (that is, repetitive tasks with short cycles) have been identified as risk factors for neck and shoulder pain. Psychological factors and personality type may be determinants of muscle tension and the development of myofascial pain.

Piece work is associated with neck and arm disorders when compared with work paid by the hour. This effect may be due to an increased work pace in addition to high psychological demand and low control in the work situation. Management style, in terms of social support to employees, is claimed to be associated with reporting of neck and shoulder symptoms. Social support from management obviously affects turnover of workers and sick leave.

Task invariability

It used to be argued that to prevent work related musculoskeletal disorders it was necessary to minimise the load that workers were exposed to. This concept has led to the creation of jobs with low external load, but some of these are still not healthy. Poor work content usually leads to a job with invariable tasks, resulting in constrained postures and a low static load for the neck and arms. Ergonomists now try to design jobs that are not only physically variable but are psychologically variable and stimulating.

The health problems caused by task invariability may be due to prolonged static contraction of the trapezius muscle during work or daily activity resulting in an overload of type I muscle fibres, which might explain neck myalgia. At a low level of muscle contraction, the low threshold motor units (type I fibres) are used. A low static contraction during work may result in a recruitment pattern in which only the type I muscle fibres are used, causing selective fatigue of motor units and damage to the type I fibres. Biopsies of the trapezius muscle from patients with work related trapezius myalgia show enlarged type I fibres and a reduced ratio of area of type I fibres to capillary area.

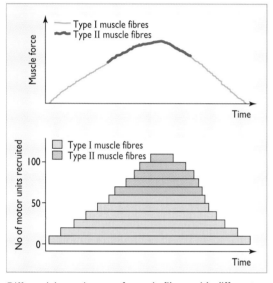

Differential recruitment of muscle fibres with different levels of contraction. At low level static contraction, only type I muscle fibres may be recruited, leading to their selective fatigue and damage.

Individual susceptibility to musculoskeletal disorders

Age
- For most musculoskeletal disorders, risk increases with age

Sex
- Among both the general population and industrial workers, women have a higher incidence of carpal tunnel syndrome and muscular pain in the neck and shoulder than men
- Whether this is due to genetic factors or to different exposures at work and at home is not clear

Anatomical differences or malformations
- A rough surface and sharp edge of the intertubercular sulcus on the humeral head increase wear on the tendon of the long head of biceps muscle, which may make a person more prone to biceps tendinitis
- A cervical rib is a common cause of neurogenic thoracic outlet syndrome: a repetitive task may be the occupational exposure that triggers clinical disease
- Width of carpal tunnel has been proposed as a risk factor for carpal tunnel syndrome, but there is no consensus

Individual susceptibility

Individuals may have increased vulnerability to injury because of disease, genetic factors, or lack of fitness. This individual susceptibility may result in a lower than normal threshold for a given exposure to cause a work related musculoskeletal disorder. Furthermore, exposure may trigger symptoms early and at an unusual location because of local strain in a person with a preclinical systemic disease. For example, a worker exposed to repetitive flexion in the shoulder developed tendinitis one year before developing rheumatoid arthritis. An electrician exposed to repetitive power grips and vibration developed symptoms and signs of carpal tunnel syndrome—at surgery, these were found to be due to amyloidosis.

For work related musculoskeletal disorders, individual factors usually have a low magnitude of risk compared with relevant ergonomic factors.

Prevention and management

Management of work related neck and arm disorders

Clinical management
- Non-steroidal anti-inflammatory drugs can reduce pain and inflammation
- Acupuncture can be used to reduce pain
- Corticosteroids – A single subacromial injection of corticosteroid mixed with local anaesthetic may cure a shoulder tendinitis. For tennis elbow and carpal tunnel syndrome, corticosteroids should be used by specialists only
- Heparin (15000 IU/day in a single intravenous dose) given for three to four days is effective treatment for acute crepitating peritendinitis
- Surgery – Surgical division of the carpal ligament is the first choice of treatment for carpal tunnel syndrome. For chronic severe shoulder tendinitis, surgical removal of the lateral part of the acromion may relieve pain at night
- Splints – Whether splints should be used to treat early hand and wrist tendinitis and carpal tunnel syndrome is still debatable

Modifications to working environment
- Job analysis – To assess work relatedness of a patient's symptoms it is necessary to evaluate posture, motion, handling of loads, psychological and social factors, and task invariability
- Job redesign – Job enlargement to reduce duration and frequency of stressful postures and load handling. Job enrichment to reduce poor work content and task invariability. Introduce new layout of workplace and technical aids
- Technique training – Ergonomists and supervisors can improve working technique to reduce stressors of postures, motion and load handling
- Rests and breaks should be organised to allow recovery

The overall objective of management is to get a healthy patient and an early return to work by medical means and by modifying the patient's working environment.

Clinical treatment should be targeted towards relieving any pain and inflammation and restoring a patient's range of movement. Physical conditioning by strength and aerobic training may reduce pain and increase a patient's work capacity, while psychological conditioning by stress management techniques may increase a person's ability to cope with work related stressors.

Patients should be encouraged to remain at work. Sick leave may develop into chronic disability. Try to find work tasks that the patient can perform at least on a part time basis. Otherwise make sure the patient has contact with the workplace at least once a week. Time off work is a powerful predictor of disability pension.

"RSI"

Principles of managing hand and arm pain in keyboard operators

- Exclude clear pathological causes such as carpal tunnel syndrome
- Reassure patient that the condition is curable
- Keep patient at work if possible but away from keyboard work if necessary
- Monitor patient's progress with regular follow up
- When symptoms have subsided advise gradual reintroduction of precipitating factors
- Explore psychological profile, including attitudes to work and support from management and colleagues
- Liaise with patient's workplace, if possible with an occupational physician or nurse
- Ensure that workstation ergonomics have been evaluated and are satisfactory and that the patient has been taught to use the equipment properly and has the right glasses
- Inquire about variation of work tasks, work intensity, and whether there are rules or opportunities for breaks from keyboard work or job rotation
- Hospital admission is rarely needed, and specialised physiotherapy is of dubious benefit
- Those few patients who do not respond to this multidisciplinary management may eventually have to be trained to use voice activated word processors, etc

In the middle and late 1980s there was an epidemic of compensation claims for so called RSI—work related pain of the arm and wrist—from keyboard operators in Australia. This coincided with the widespread replacement of typewriters with computer keyboards. At one extreme, this was thought to be a genuine overuse syndrome, while, at the other, it was regarded as mass hysteria with an element of bandwagoning. RSI also appeared in other countries, while its incidence progressively declined in Australia, where claims had grown to such a size that the government changed the compensation system so that symptoms associated with using keyboards were no longer compensated.

A country's compensation system has a great effect on the reporting and control of work related disorders. In Sweden there has been a substantial decrease in reported work related diseases, probably due to an increased demand for evidence of work relatedness before compensation is approved. This conjecture is supported by statistics showing that rates of reported work related musculoskeletal symptoms in national surveys are constant. A generous compensation system can lead to patients becoming medicalised and lacking the motivation to attempt rehabilitation. However, a compensation system that facilitates reporting of work related disorders allows early identification of hazards that may constitute a serious risk to a workforce.

The existence of RSI as a clinical entity has been challenged medically and legally. Many sufferers have won compensation, but very few have secured damages by means of civil litigation—almost all claims are settled out of court. The diagnosis of RSI (a completely unsatisfactory term as explained earlier) is usually one of exclusion, there being, by definition, no physical signs. Whatever the true nature of the condition, almost every doctor will see patients who relate their pain syndrome to keyboard work, and management is seldom easy or straightforward. Ideally, it should be multidisciplinary.

Key references

- Aarås A. The impact of ergonomic intervention on individual health and corporate prosperity in a telecommunications environment. *Ergonomics* 1994;**37**:1679–96
- Bongers PM, de Winter CR, Kompier MA, Hildebranndt VH. Psychosocial factors at work and musculoskeletal disease. *Scand J Work Environ Health* 1993; **19**:297–312
- Gerr F, Letz R, Landrigan PJ. Upper-extremity musculoskeletal disorders of occupational origin. *Ann Rev Publ Health* 1991;**12**:543–66
- Kuorinka I, Forcier L, eds. *Work related musculoskeletal disorders (WMSDs): a reference book for prevention*. London: Taylor and Francis, 1995
- Hagberg M. Neck and shoulder disorders. In: Rosenstock L, Cullen MR, eds. *Textbook of occupational and environmental medicine*. Philadelphia, PA: W B Saunders, 1994: 356–64

6 OCCUPATIONAL DERMATITIS

Ian R White

Sheeted eczema over dorsal aspect of hand and up forearm due to allergic contact dermatitis to a carbamate accelerator in protective rubber gloves.

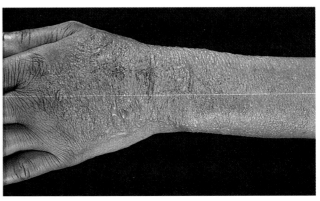

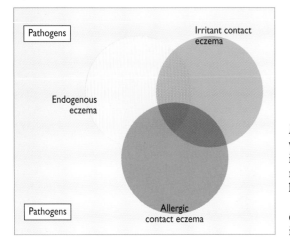

Dermatitis may be endogenous or exogenous, or a combination of these, and may be aggravated by pathogens.

Dermatitis of occupational cause may be suspected when:

- Dermatitis first occurred while employed
- There is a history of aggravation by work
- There may be, at least initially, improvement (or clearance) when not at work
- There is exposure to irritant factors or potential allergens
- Work is in an "at risk" occupation

Many dermatoses may have occupational relevance, but the overwhelming majority are dermatitic. In current terminology "dermatitis" is used synonymously with "eczema" to describe inflammatory reactions in the skin with a particular spectrum of clinical and histopathological characteristics.

A dermatitis may be entirely endogenous (constitutional) or be entirely exogenous (contact). Exogenous dermatitis may be caused by irritant or allergic contact reactions. A dermatitis often has a multifactorial aetiology and may be aggravated by the presence of pathogens such as *Staphylococcus aureus*. When considering a hand eczema it is always worth investigating the possible role of contributory factors and assessing the importance of these. Atopic hand eczema is a common example of an endogenous eczema in which exogenous factors normally compound the situation.

An occupational dermatitis is one where the inflammatory reaction is caused entirely by occupational contact factors or where such agents are partly responsible by contributing to the reaction on compromised skin. In most cases occupationally related dermatitis affects the hands alone, though there may be spread onto the forearms. Occasionally, the face may be the prime site of inflammation (for example, with airborne contact factors), and other sites may be affected.

Irritant contact dermatitis

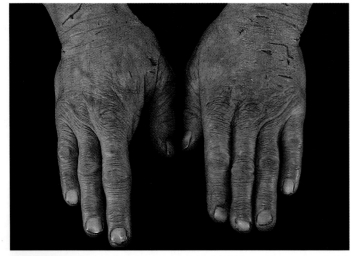

Lichenified and fissured eczema on hands of bricklayer due to chronic irritant contact dermatitis. Patch tests were negative, and he was not sensitive to chromate.

Irritant contact dermatitis is caused by direct chemical or physical damage to the skin. Everyone is susceptible to the development of an irritant contact dermatitis if exposure to an irritant (toxic) agent is sufficient. It occurs particularly where the stratum corneum is thinnest. Hence, it is often seen in the finger webs and back of the hands rather than the palms.

Examples of common irritants

- "Wet work"
- Solvents
- Detergents
- Soluble coolants
- Vegetable juices
- Wet cement

With all of above, skin may be "hit" at several target sites, causing damage by several mechanisms

---

20

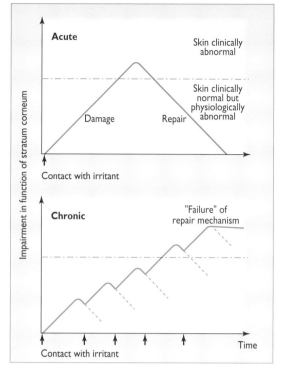

Development of acute and chronic irritant contact dermatitis

There are two main types of irritant contact dermatitis—acute and chronic. The acute form occurs after exposure to an agent or agents causing early impairment in the function of the stratum corneum and an inflammatory reaction. The chronic form follows repeated exposure to the same or different factors causing cumulative damage until an inflammatory reaction ensues that persists even after further exposure is stopped. People with a history of atopic eczema, especially atopic hand eczema, are at particular risk of developing a chronic irritant contact dermatitis. This chronic dermatitis is particularly observed in jobs that include "wet work."

Irritant contact dermatitis

Acute
- Severity of reaction depends on dose of irritant agent
- Chapping can be considered a minor form and a chemical burn (such as cement burn) an extreme event
- Intermediate eczematous reactions are common, and minor reactions are very common
- It may occur on the face—for example, low humidity occupational dermatosis, airborne irritant vapours
- Once irritant factors have been removed, resolution is usually spontaneous without important sequelae

Chronic
- Persistent dermatitis, the most common cause of continued disability from occupational skin disease
- Problem continues for long periods even with avoidance of aggravating factors
- Re-exposure to even minor irritant factors can cause rapid flare
- Even after apparent healing there may be an indefinitely increased susceptibility to recurrence of dermatitis after exposure to irritants

---

Allergic contact dermatitis

Common occupational allergens
- Rubber accelerating chemicals—such as thiurams, carbamates, mercaptobenzothiazole
- Biocides — such as formaldehyde, isothiazolinones
- Hairdressing chemicals — such as thioglycolates, *p*-phenylendiamine
- Epoxy resin monomers
- Chromate
- Plant allergens—such as sesquiterpene lactones

Allergic contact dermatitis is a manifestation of a type IV hypersensitivity reaction. The dermatitis develops at the site of skin contact with the allergen. Secondary spread may occur. Contaminated hands may spread the allergen to previously unexposed sites. Trivial ot occult contact with an allergen may result in a persistence of a dermatitis. Some allergens are essentially ubiquitous—for example, formaldehyde and sesquiterpene lactones.

There are two phases to the presentation of an allergic contact reaction: induction, during which the state of hypersensitivity to a molecule is acquired, and elicitation, whereby an eczematous reaction follows from subsequent exposure to the substance. Even with potent experimental allergens there is a minimum period of about 10 days from first exposure to the immunological acquisition of hypersensitivity. The probability of developing hypersensitivity depends on the sensitising capacity of the chemical and exposure to it. Most potential allergens in the domestic and industrial market have low intrinsic potential for sensitisation, with the important exception of some biocides. Contact allergens tend to be of low molecular weight (< 600) and capable of forming covalent bonds with carrier proteins in the skin.

It is not yet possible to determine an individual's susceptibility to developing contact allergy. Hypersensitivity is specific to a particular molecule or to molecules bearing similar allergenic sites. Although hypersensitivity may eventually be lost, the state should be considered to last indefinitely.

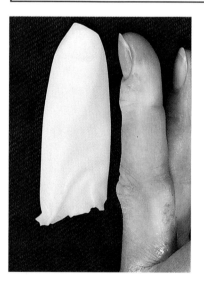

Immediate contact reaction to latex protein in examination gloves. Type I reactions to latex protein are of growing concern.

Rubber latex protein sensitivity

Of concern is the increasing occurrence of immediate type I hypersensitivity to proteins present in gloves made from natural rubber latex. The problem is seen principally among health workers, but people in other industries where examination gloves are used are also at risk. The Medical Devices Agency has published a bulletin describing the problem.[1]

Primary prevention involves the use of non-powdered gloves with very low protein residues. Affected people need to be provided with synthetic alternatives to rubber.

Sensitisation to latex gloves
- Affected people are usually atopic
- Presentation may be localised urticarial reaction at sites of skin contact or may be respiratory symptoms when starch powdered gloves have been used
- Has become an important cause of occupational morbidity in some groups—for example, dental students
- Anaphylaxis is possible with appropriate exposure
- Definitive demonstration of hypersensitivity can be made by prick testing with water soluble proteins

Management of occupational dermatitis

Patterns of hand dermatitis

- From distribution and morphology of dermatitis on hands, it is not possible to be definitive about aetiology
- Thus, vesicular hand dermatitis with classic endogenous distribution may be mimicked by allergic contact dermatitis to isothiazolinone biocides or chromate sensitivity
- It is a major error to rely on patterns of hand dermatitis alone in making a diagnosis

Patch testing

- Properly performed, it requires expertise, time, and proper facilities
- Difficult to undertake adequately in the workplace – there are no shortcuts
- Primarily a hospital based procedure
- Should be performed only by those with proper training who
    Can prescribe an appropriately comprehensive screen
    Know what not to test
    Know what to dilute for testing
    Can competently read the reactions
    Can give authoritative advice after interpreting the reactions

Anyone can patch test, but few do it well—if you don't know how to do it, don't do it

Preventing occupational dermatitis

- Primary prevention is aimed at providing appropriate information and protection
- Employer and employee should be aware of potential risks of exposure
- Education of need for good occupational hygiene
- Adequate provision of suitable and effective means of reducing exposure
- Awareness of limitations of personal protection devices

Key reference

- Medical Devices Agency. *Latex sensitisation in the health care setting (use of latex gloves)* London: MDA, April 1996. (Device bulletin MDA DB 9601.)

Assessment

Understanding the patient's job is necessary. A job title is not sufficient for this understanding; the question to be asked is not "What do you do?" but "What exactly do you do and how do you do it?" The title "engineer" can mean anything from a desk bound professional to a lathe worker exposed to soluble coolants. From a good job description it may be possible to estimate sources of excessive contact with potential irritant contact factors or with allergens. Data sheets may be helpful in this evaluation, but the information that they contain is often superficial and is only what is needed to meet regulatory requirements. A site visit—watching the patient working—may be necessary.

The history of the dermatitis may provide clues as to the aetiology. Irritant contact dermatitis may occur as an "epidemic" in a workplace if hygiene has failed, while allergic contact dermatitis is usually sporadic.

Evaluation of contact factors—The evaluation of irritant factors is always subjective. Evaluation of allergic contact factors is objective and is provided only by diagnostic patch tests. Properly performed, patch tests will show the presence or absence of important allergens. Patch testing is the only method for the objective evaluation of a dermatitis. There are major pitfalls in the use of this essential tool—proper training and experience are essential if it is to provide valid results.

A competent assessment requires all of the above followed by recommendations on reducing or stopping exposure to the offending agent and similar ones.

Diagnosis

The diagnosis of an occupational dermatitis should describe thoroughly the nature of the condition, including any endogenous or aggravating factors. A medical record in a patient's notes of "Works in a factory, contact dermatitis 2/52" is inadequate as a description of an important disease process, and it could have profound implications for the patient's concept of the problem and employment. Delays in diagnosis that result in continued exposure to relevant irritants or allergens can adversely affect the prognosis.

Early referral to an appropriate dermatology department is vital for a full assessment of a suspected occupational dermatitis. Improper assessment can have a devastating effect on a patient's prospects for future employment, with important medicolegal implications. If in doubt, refer. Also consider contacting the patient's occupational health department if there is one.

7 OCCUPATIONAL INFECTIONS

David Snashall

Occupational groups at risk of infections contracted at work

- Veterinary surgeons – leptospirosis, Q fever
- Farm workers – ringworm, leptospirosis, orf, tetanus, perhaps bovine spongiform encephalopathy
- Poultry workers – ornithosis, histoplasmosis, Newcastle disease
- Health workers – hepatitis, HIV
- Construction workers – tetanus
- Butchers and abattoir workers – *Streptococcus suis*, Q fever
- Forestry workers – Lyme disease
- Engineering workers – skin infection
- Overseas workers returning home – tropical diseases, brucellosis, anthrax

Specific infections due to work are not common, but some systemic ones are serious and easy to miss unless there is a high index of suspicion. Carefully taking a patient's occupational history may reveal the diagnosis for an unusual illness. Superficial infections are less serious but may be difficult to diagnose and treat and can be transmitted to others. Some infections may cause an allergic response (such as farmer's lung), and endotoxins and mycotoxins can cause acute and chronic respiratory symptoms (such as mycobyssinosis in cotton workers). Like all occupational diseases, occupational infections are mostly preventable.

Some infections are included in the list of diseases prescribed under the Industrial Injuries Provisions of the Social Security Act 1975. The affected person can claim "no fault" compensation from the government if the "prescribed" disease is considered to be the result of certain kinds of work and if disability is rated at over 14%

There is a similar list of "reportable" diseases, some of them infectious, caused by work, and it is the duty of the employer (often advised by the doctor who diagnoses the disease) to report them under the RIDDOR regulations to the Health and Safety Executive or, sometimes, to the local environmental health department. They used to be called "notifiable" occupational diseases. The name changed in 1980, and they should be distinguished from those infectious diseases that are notifiable under the Public Health Acts. Later this year CCDCs will start reporting occupational infections, publishing the numbers quarterly.

Employers are also bound to comply with the COSHH regulations when there is a risk of infectious disease associated with work. This demands a formal assessment of risk and the institution of precautions.

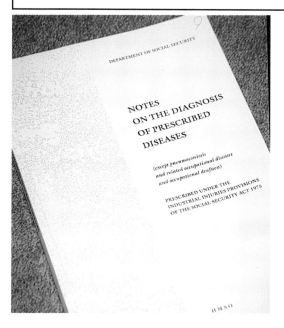

Specific infections

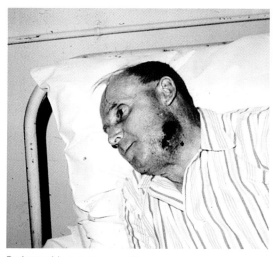

Patient with cutaneous anthrax.

Anthrax

This is now rare in Britain and occurs in people who come into contact with animals infected with anthrax or who deal with animal products or residues (usually from abroad) that are contaminated with anthrax spores. The causative agent is *Bacillus anthracis*, and the disease usually presents as a black pustule or eschar on the skin at the site of primary infection. If not treated, this form of cutaneous anthrax leads to toxaemia and death. The organism is usually sensitive to penicillin. People who are most commonly affected are veterinary surgeons, butchers, slaughterers, and farm workers.

More severe forms of the disease—pulmonary or gastrointestinal—are due to the inhalation or ingestion of anthrax spores. "Wool sorter's disease," the pulmonary form, is rapidly fatal and used to be seen in factories that dealt with imported wool or hides. Unsterilised bone meal used as a fertiliser is another source. Pulmonary anthrax remains a potential agent for germ warfare.

One or two cases of cutaneous anthrax have been notified annually since 1982
There have been no cases of wool sorter's disease in Britain since the 1930s. By contrast, Turkey, for example, reports 350 cases a year

Occupational infections

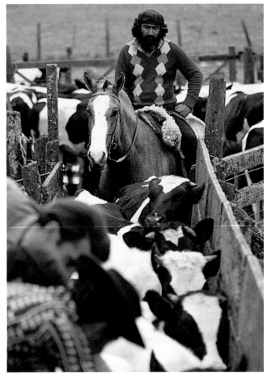

Farm workers are at increased risk of catching animal borne diseases.

Glanders and ankylostomiasis

These two infections no longer occur in Britain but may be imported from abroad. Glanders is systemic infection with *Actinobacillus mallei*, caught from horses. Ankylostomiasis is infection with hookworms of the genus *Ancylostoma*. These nematodes can survive and be transmitted during mining work and were once common in Cornish tin mines. The disease remains common in the tropics.

Brucellosis

Infection with *Brucella abortus*, which causes undulant fever, is also now a rarity in Britain due to the Ministry of Agriculture's crusade over the past 20 years to eradicate the disease in cattle by slaughtering and inoculation. Sufferers were usually farm workers and vets, with an occasional laboratory acquired infection. Infection with *B abortus* (from cattle), *B melitensis* (from sheep and goats), and *B suis* (from pigs) is still common in many developing countries and should be suspected in people such as overseas aid workers in veterinary or farming jobs who return to Britain with fever and lymphadenopathy. It may also occur in foreign travellers who have consumed unpasteurised milk products.

Leptospirosis

Weil's disease, caused by *Leptospira icterohaemorrhagiae*, was once an important disease of canal and sewage workers but is now rare as an occupational disease. It is caught, usually percutaneously, by exposure to leptospires in rat's urine and typically presents as a high fever, headache, muscular pains, and vomiting with jaundice, bleeding disorders, hepatosplenomegaly, and renal failure. Workers who may be exposed to leptospires usually carry a card provided by their employer to show to their doctor if they develop such symptoms.

Infection with a variety of other leptospires is much more common, particularly infection with *L hebdomadis* serovariant Hardjo, which causes cattle associated leptospirosis (CAL). This condition is likely to be seen in dairy workers, vets, etc. It is also transmitted via urine and presents as a flu-like illness, sometimes with mental confusion, and will run for months unless treated with antibiotics.

Water associated leptospiroses (Weil's disease and canicola fever) are also a recognised hazard for people indulging in water sports, especially canoeists. Most British rivers and canals carry pathogenic leptospires. Protective clothing, including gloves, is the main preventive measure, and early recognition that a fever of unknown origin could be leptospirosis will improve the final outcome.

Tuberculosis

As an occupationally acquired infection, tuberculosis mainly occurs in health workers. With the recent increase in cases of pulmonary tuberculosis worldwide and in certain communities in Britain, extra vigilance may be required. Laboratory workers used to face the highest risk, but this has now declined because of strict rules about processing tuberculous materials and the development of safe working practices. Necropsy workers also have specific codes that they should follow when dealing with possibly tuberculous cases. Tuberculosis is no longer a hazard in British agricultural industry.

To protect health workers against tuberculosis, their immune status should be checked when they start work or studies. A definite BCG vaccination scar obviates the need for tuberculin testing. Those with poor tuberculin reactivity should be vaccinated with BCG. Routine chest *x* ray examinations for health workers are no longer considered necessary, either at recruitment or periodically thereafter. Health workers born overseas often have strongly positive tuberculin reactions, but this is generally less important than finding a strongly positive reaction in a British born person. Such a finding at recruitment may require further investigations, as it may in a person who has recently come from a country where tuberculosis is common.

Education of staff about the symptoms of tuberculosis is important, especially if they are likely to be dealing with patients who may have as yet undiagnosed pulmonary tuberculosis. Symptoms—coughing, sweats, and weight loss—must be investigated in the usual way.

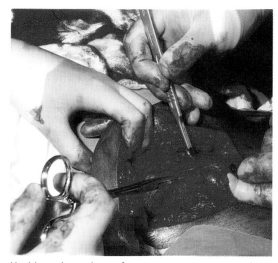
Health workers who perform exposure prone procedures should be vaccinated against hepatitis B.

Viral hepatitis

Hepatitis B and C are mainly a risk to health workers, although others such as prison warders and police officers may be exposed to hepatitis, usually blood transmitted. Hepatitis A, mainly spread by the faecal-oral route, has been transmitted by food handling procedures. There is a theoretical risk to sewage workers and hospital laboratory staff, but no excess numbers of cases have been recorded in these occupations.

Infection of health care workers may be with hepatitis A, B, or C or with various other agents—Epstein-Barr virus, cytomegalovirus, etc. One of the most important of these is hepatitis B, which represents a substantial risk to health workers, especially if they perform invasive or "exposure prone" procedures or if they work abroad in countries where the prevalence of the disease is high. Immunisation against hepatitis B is available, remarkably effective, and becoming cheaper. All medical students should be vaccinated before they start clinical work, as should other health workers, including dentists, who may be exposed to blood and body fluids, especially in uncontrolled circumstances such as accident and emergency work. It is doubtful whether the risk to other occupational groups warrants vaccination.

Recent guidelines from the Department of Health have emphasised the importance of vaccination against hepatitis B to protect health workers and their patients. Workers who perform exposure prone procedures (essentially deep surgery, blind needling, and dentistry) should, if they are not naturally immune or successfully vaccinated, be tested to exclude carriage of hepatitis B virus. If positive, they should be offered treatment or redeployed to safer work if they remain infectious. The incidence of hepatitis B in health workers will decline as these procedures are taken up.

Chronic carriers of hepatitis B e antigen are infectious via their blood and body fluids and need only avoid performing exposure prone operations. They require expert confidential counselling about sexual contacts and possible redeployment and retraining. After a needlestick injury, a risk assessment must be made and a blood sample for serology may be required—for hepatitis B and, when relevant, for HIV and hepatitis C.

Both hepatitis B and C have been transmitted from patients to health workers. No vaccine against hepatitis C has yet been developed; health workers who have transmitted the disease should be barred from performing exposure prone procedures. Treatment with interferon alfa should be considered for chronic carriers of hepatitis B or C antigens.

HIV infection

The HIV virus is transmitted in the same way as hepatitis B but with much greater difficulty. So far as is known (a transmission rate of 0·3% has been suggested) health workers have rarely been affected in this country. There are, however, around 60 reports worldwide of health workers who have apparently acquired HIV infection from professional contact with patients. These patients have usually been suffering from frank AIDS and a quantity of blood or other body fluid has been inoculated into the health workers, with subsequent seroconversion. Health care workers abroad may be at greater risk.

Protective measures are the same as for hepatitis B—use of universal precautions in handling blood and body fluids, care with needles, no resheathing of hollow needles, proper disposal of sharps, prompt first aid after sharps injuries, and proper reporting of such injuries.

The use of zidovudine as post-exposure prophylaxis is still controversial. The use of newer antiviral drugs in combination has also been recommended. To be effective, these drugs must be administered rapidly—within an hour of exposure if possible. A local policy on their use should be developed. Health workers who have suffered an injury that might have transmitted HIV need expert counselling and follow up testing for HIV antibody, preferably by an occupational health department or a doctor with experience of HIV infection.

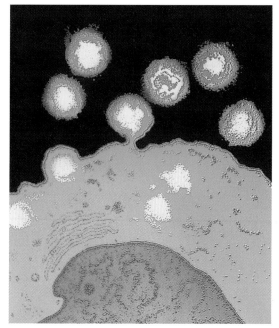
Enhanced, false colour electron micrograph showing HIV budding out of infected human T lymphocyte.

Disease spread from farm animals

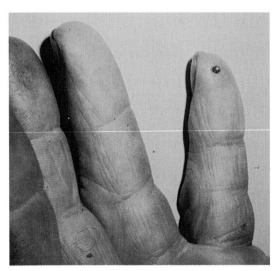

Typical painless blister of orf.

Streptococcus suis causes an infection characterised by septicaemia, meningitis, possibly arthritis, pharyngitis, and diarrhoea. It is transmitted from seemingly healthy pigs and their carcases and thus may be a problem for butchers and slaughterers as well as pig breeders.

Avian chlamydiosis (ornithosis, psittacosis) usually presents as an atypical pneumonia and occurs when workers with turkeys, ducks, chickens, pigeons, and exotic birds inhale the dust of dried excreta or feathers. Vets, quarantine station workers, pet shop owners, and poultry workers may be affected.

Ovine chlamydiosis presents as an acute flu-like illness in vets, agricultural workers, shepherds, and abattoir workers who handle infected sheep. Abortion may occur in pregnant women.

Q fever due to *Coxiella burnetii* causes a flu-like illness with possible pneumonia, pericarditis, myocarditis, and encephalitis. The chronic form may affect the aortic valve. It is usually caught from sheep, cattle, or goats, particularly from contact with placentas or unpasteurised milk.

Newcastle disease from fowls can also cause a flu-like illness or conjunctivitis.

Histoplasmosis, due to inhalation of spores of the fungus *Histoplasma capsulatum,* causes respiratory symptoms and may be caught from chicken manure.

Skin infections – Ringworm can be transmitted from cattle and horses. Orf (contagious pustular dermatitis) is a self limiting disease caught from sheep and usually presents on the hands as painless blisters. Hydatid disease is now rare in Britain but is sometimes found in rural communities.

Non-agricultural diseases

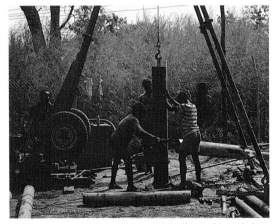

Workers in forested areas are at risk of acquiring viral haemorrhagic fevers.

The re-use of cutting oils in engineering works can lead to oil mists being contaminated with bacteria and fungi, and these have been implicated in various types of skin infection. Deep sea divers who use saturation techniques—in which they remain under increased barometric pressure for some weeks—are prone to otitis externa, especially with *Pseudomonas* species. Legionellosis is sometimes occupationally acquired (see chapter on building related illnesses).

Viral haemorrhagic fevers, even yellow fever, can be occupational because they tend to be transmitted to agricultural or forest workers when they are clearing crops or trees. The diseases are sometimes imported and transmitted to health workers—Lassa fever, for example.

Forest workers may be at increased risk of Lyme disease. A bite from an infected tick transmits the causative organism *Borrellia burgdorferi.* Early symptoms are a red area around the bite, fever, joint pains, and headache. A variety of symptoms may supervene if the disease is not rapidly recognised and treated with antibiotics.

Immunisations

Occupations that require specific immunisations

- Health workers – vaccination against rubella, hepatitis B, tuberculosis (BCG vaccine), and possibly chicken pox
- Construction workers, etc – vaccination against tetanus
- Agricultural workers – vaccination against tetanus.
- Veterinary surgeons – vaccination against tetanus and possibly rabies

The micrograph of budding HIV was produced by Chris Bjornberg and is reproduced with permission of Science Photo Library.

Because of their increased risk of infection, workers in certain occupations need specific immunisations.

Influenza vaccination is heavily advertised every year but is not indicated for healthy young workers, and the immunisation itself can cause some morbidity. Its efficacy in a particular outbreak is difficult to predict, and it is unlikely to reduce levels of absence attributable to sickness. It should be retained for people with chronic disease, for whom an attack of flu would be disastrous.

There is much regional variation in occupationally acquired infections. International travel has increased the rate of imported disease to Britain. Workers may go into areas where tourists do not visit and often experience worse conditions. They are often abroad for longer periods of time. Malaria still probably presents the commonest and most serious of such infections (see *ABC of Healthy Travel*).

8 OCCUPATIONAL CANCERS

Charles Veys

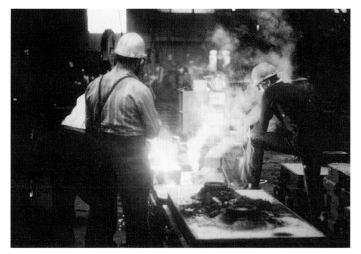

Foundry workers may be exposed to a complex mixture of carcinogenic agents in fumes.

The first report of cancer caused by occupational exposure was in 1775 by Percival Pott, a British surgeon who described scrotal cancer in boy chimney sweeps. A century later, in 1895, Rehn, a German surgeon working in Frankfurt, treated a cluster of three cases of bladder cancer in workers at a local factory producing aniline dyestuffs from coal tar.

Occupational cancer is any malignancy wholly or partly caused by exposures at the workplace or in occupation. Such exposure may be to a particular chemical (such as β-naphthylamine), a physical agent (such as ionising radiation or a fibre like asbestos), a biological agent (such as hepatitis B virus), or an industrial process in which the specific carcinogen may elude precise definition (such as coke production).

Of all the occupationally related diseases, cancer evokes particular concern and strong emotions, because of the opportunity afforded for attribution, blame, and compensation. On the other hand, occupational cancers have unique potential for prevention.

About 4% of all cancer deaths in people aged over 15 years may have an occupational cause. This translates into over 3000 male deaths in England and Wales from potentially preventable malignancies. The proportion occurring in women is probably less because of their lower potential for exposure.

The International Agency for Research on Cancer (IARC) was set up within the World Health Organisation in 1971 to assess whether individual agents, mixtures, and occupational exposures have carcinogenic potential for humans. Since 1972 the agency has published 66 monographs covering more than 700 such evaluations. Today, some 65 agents and occupational environments are regarded by IARC as established human carcinogens. Over 50 are listed as probably carcinogenic, and about 300 are thought to be possibly carcinogenic.

Characteristics of occupational cancer

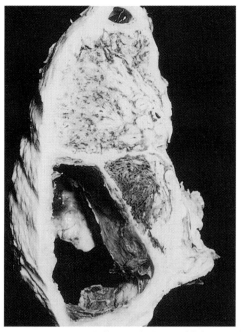

Thick walled mesothelioma of pleura with haemorrhagic cavitation in a former insulation worker.

Mechanisms

Cancer induction is a complex multistage process in which nuclear damage occurs at an early stage.

Genotoxic (DNA reactive) carcinogens interact with and alter DNA.

Epigenetic carcinogens act more directly on the cell itself, through hormonal imbalances, immunological effects, or promoter activity, to cause abnormal cell proliferation and chromosomal aberrations that affect gene expression.

Site of cancers

The target organ is usually singular and site specific, but not necessarily so. In Britain the most commonly affected sites are the lung and mesothelium ($\sim 75\%$), bladder ($\sim 10\%$), and skin ($< 1\%$), with the haemopoietic system, nasal cavities, larynx, and liver much less affected.

Natural course of cancers

Occupationally related cancers are characterised by a long latent period—that is, the time between first exposure to the causative agent and presentation of the tumour. This latency is not usually less than 10-15 years and can be much longer—40-50 years in the case of some asbestos related mesotheliomas. Thus, presentation can be in retirement rather than while still at work.

An occupationally related tumour does not differ substantially, either pathologically or clinically, from its "naturally occurring" counterpart.

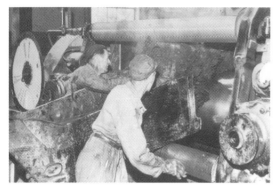
Rubber workers in mill room.

Effective dose of carcinogen

There is probably a minimal threshold dose as well as a clear dose-response relation influencing the occurrence of cancers. For example, all workers involved in distilling β-naphthylamine eventually developed tumours of the urothelial tract, whereas only 4% of rubber mill workers—who were exposed to β-naphthylamine contaminating an antioxidant (at 0.25%) used in making tyres and inner tubes—developed bladder cancer over a 30 year follow up. Studies indicate that susceptibility to occupational carcinogens is greater when the exposure occurs at younger ages.

Recognition and diagnosis

Diagnosis of work related cancer is assisted by

- Detailed lifelong occupational history
- Comparison with a check list of recognised causal associations
- Search for additional clues:
  Shift to a younger age
  Presence of signal tumours
  Other cases and "clusters"
  Long latency
  Absence of anticipated aetiologies
  Unusual histology or site
- Confirmation of requisite exposure

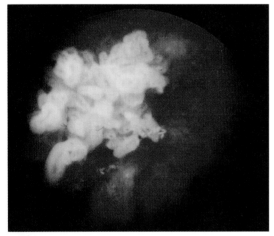
Cystoscopic view of papillary carcinoma of the bladder in a 47 year old rubber worker.

For a group of workers, occupational cancer is evidenced by a clear excess of cancers over what would normally be expected. However, it is not possible to distinguish individual tumours that were actually caused by the occupational exposure from those that would have occurred anyway. Furthermore, some common malignancies that can be work related also have a well recognised and predominant aetiology related to other agents, diet, or lifestyle (for example, lung cancer from smoking). There are, however, some features which may help to distinguish occupational cancers from those not related to work.

History taking—Taking a patient's occupational history (that is, since leaving school until retirement or the present) is of paramount importance. It should be defined in detail and sequentially. For example, a holiday job in a factory that lasted only a few months could easily be overlooked, but it may have involved delagging a boiler or handling sacks of asbestos waste.

Signal tumours—Several uncommon cancers are associated with particular occupations. Thus, an angiosarcoma of the liver may indicate past exposure to vinyl chloride monomer in the production of polyvinyl chloride (PVC); a laryngeal tumour may have derived from exposure to the fumes of strong acids as well as from cigarette smoke; a nasal cancer may have resulted from exposure to dusts from hardwood in furniture manufacture. These less common cancers are sometimes called signal tumours because they should always alert a doctor to a possible occupational aetiology.

Age—A younger age at presentation with cancer may suggest an occupational influence. For example, a tumour of the urothelial tract presenting in anyone under the age of 50 years should always arouse suspicion.

Patients' information—Patients may speak of a "cluster" of cancer cases at work or may have worked in an industry or job for which a warning leaflet has been issued.

Prevention

Action for primary prevention of occupational cancers

- Recognising presence of hazards and risks
- Educating management and workforce
- Eliminating exposure by substitution and automation
- Reducing exposure by engineering controls (such as local exhaust ventilation and enclosure), changes in handling, and altering physical form in processing
- Monitoring exposure and maintaining plant
- Protecting workers by means of personal protective equipment
- Limiting access
- Providing adequate facilities for showering, washing, and changing
- Legislative provisions

Secondary prevention of occupational cancer is helped by screening tests and medical surveillance—for example, exfoliative urinary cytology and skin inspections

Primary prevention of occupationally related cancers depends essentially on educating employers and employees – firstly, about recognising that there is a risk, and then about the practical steps that can be taken to eliminate or reduce exposure and to protect operators. Modern legislation now directs these educational and practical measures.

Secondary prevention – Screening procedures can be used if they might help with earlier diagnosis (for example, exfoliative urinary cytology), but the final outcome may not necessarily be altered. Once initiated, such surveillance must be lifelong or until old age or other serious intercurrent illness intervenes. Routine skin inspections are a very effective method of secondary prevention for cutaneous cancers of occupational origin because of the excellent prognosis afforded by treatment.

Legislation and statutory compensation

Main legislative provisions in the United Kingdom
- Control of Substances Hazaeous to Health (COSHH) Regulations 1994 and associated ACOP on the Control of Carcinogens
- European Commission Carcinogens Directive (90/934/EEC)
- Chemicals (Hazard Information and Packaging) Regulations 1993 (CHIP)
- Ionising Radiation Regulations (1985)
- Control of Asbestos at Work Regulations (1988).
- Reporting of Injuries, Diseases and Dangerous Occurrences Regulations 1995 (RIDDOR)

Essential legislative provisions in Britain and the European Community are comprehensive. Ten types of cancer are prescribed diseases, which means that sufferers can claim social security benefits. Some cancers are also notifiable under the RIDDOR regulations. In 1993 the 713 new cases of occupational cancer prescribed under the various industrial injuries benefit schemes (mesothelioma 608 cases, asbestos related lung cancer 72, bladder cancer 26, others 7) almost certainly considerably underrepresented the true picture.

Specific carcinogens

Metalliferous carcinogens

Agent	Target organ
● Arsenic	Lung, skin
● Beryllium	Lung
● Cadmium	Lung, prostate gland
● Chromium (hexavalent)	Lung
● Nickel	Lung, nasal sinuses
● Iron in: Haematite mining (radon)	Lung
Iron and steel founding	Lung, digestive tract

Metals and metalliferous compounds

Arsenic, beryllium, cadmium, chromium (VI), nickel, and iron are considered to be proved human carcinogens, either as the metal itself or as a derivative. The risk from iron is related only to mining the base ore and is due to coincidental exposure to radon gas. In foundries, where there is concomitant exposure to several agents in a complex mix of emanating fume, the responsible agents are not clearly defined.

With all the metallic carcinogens, the lung is the main target organ, but other potential sites are the skin (arsenic), prostate gland (cadmium), and nasal sinuses (nickel), indicating the metals' pluripotential nature.

The main occupational exposures occur in the mining, smelting, founding, and refining of these metals, and less commonly in secondary industrial use.

Aromatic amine carcinogens

Agent	Target organ
● 4-Aminobiphenyl (xenylamine) and its nitro derivative ● β-naphthylamine ● Benzidine ● Auramine and magenta (in manufacture only)	Bladder predominantly, but also other parts of the urothelial tract lined by transitional cell epithelium (renal pelvis, ureter, and first part of prostatic uretha)

Recent evidence also implicates the polycyclic aromatic hydrocarbons as probable human urinary tract carcinogens, and the hardener MbOCA ($4_1,4^1$-methylene-bis-(2-chloroaniline)) is suspect

Aromatic amines

Aromatic amines are one of the best known and most studied of chemical carcinogens. The bladder is the main target organ, but any site on the urothelial tract comprised of transitional cell epithelium can be affected—that is, from the renal pelvis to the prostatic urethra. Tumours of the upper urothelial tract (renal pelvis or ureter) are very uncommon, and a cluster of these signal tumours usually heralds an underlying risk of occupational cancer. The carcinogenic potential of aromatic amines lies not in the parent compound but in a metabolite formed in the liver and excreted through the urinary system.

Occupations causally associated with urothelial tract cancers
- Dyestuffs and pigment manufacture
- Rubber workers (in tyre, tube, cable, and some general goods manufacture before 1950)
- Textile dyeing and printing
- Manufacture of some organic chemicals (such as MbOCA)
- Gas workers (in old vertical retort houses)
- Laboratory and testing work (using chromogens)
- Rodent controllers (formally using ANTU (α-naphthylthiourea))
- Painters
- Leather workers
- Manufacture of patent fuel (such as coke) and firelighters
- Tar and pitch workers (roofing and road maintenance)
- Aluminium refining

The occupations classically associated with risk from these chemicals were in the industries manufacturing chemicals and dyestuffs—a detailed study of this risk led to occupational bladder cancer becoming a prescribed disease in 1953.

Antioxidants contaminated with β-naphthylamine—one of the most potent bladder carcinogens—were used in the rubber and cable making industries until the end of 1949, when they were universally withdrawn, and they caused an excess of bladder cancer. The level of contamination was only about 0·25%, yet it almost doubled the risk for the workforce so exposed. People who started work in the rubber industry after 1951 seem to have no excess risk.

Although the presenting pathology is often that of a papillary tumour, it can range from carcinoma in situ to an advanced infiltrating lesion. At most, only about 6% of all bladder tumours registered annually are realistically work related. This contrasts with the 30–50% that can probably be attributed to tobacco smoking.

There is now increasing evidence that some polycyclic aromatic hydrocarbons can also act as urinary tract carcinogens. This is reflected in excesses seen in aluminium refiners and in painters exposed to solvents.

Occupational cancers

Asbestos

Few natural materials used in industry have been the subject of more epidemiological and pathological research than the asbestos fibre. Its association with lung cancer was finally confirmed in the middle 1950s, and with mesothelioma nearly a decade later.

In asbestos workers who have developed asbestosis the risk of lung cancer is increased at least fivefold. Smoking with concomitant exposure to asbestos also greatly increases the risk of developing lung cancer. This synergistic action is multiplicative: compared with non-smokers not exposed to asbestos, a smoker exposed to asbestos has a 75–100 times greater risk if exposure was sufficient to cause asbestosis, otherwise the risk is about 30–50 times higher. Over 40% of people with asbestosis die of lung cancer, and 10% die of mesothelioma.

Mesotheliomas, which are predominantly of the pleura (ratio of 8:1 with peritoneum), have usually been growing for 10–12 years before becoming clinically evident. Thus latency can be very long—often 30 years and sometimes up to 50 years. However, median survival from the time of initial diagnosis is usually short, some three to 12 months.

The amphibole fibres in crocidolite (blue asbestos) and amosite (brown asbestos) carry the greatest risk of causing mesothelioma, but the serpentine fibres in chrysotile (white asbestos) can also do so, especially if they contain tremolite.

Mesothelioma extending through needle biopsy tract.

In about 90% of patients with mesothelioma, close questioning will usually reveal some earlier exposure to asbestos. The prevalence of mesothelioma is increasing; it currently causes more than 1000 deaths annually in Britain, and it is no longer a rare disease. It is predicted that, by the year 2020, there will be up to 3300 deaths annually. The possible risk to neighbourhoods outside asbestos factories from discharged asbestos dust or contaminated clothing brought home should not be forgotten.

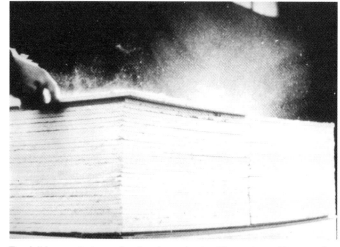
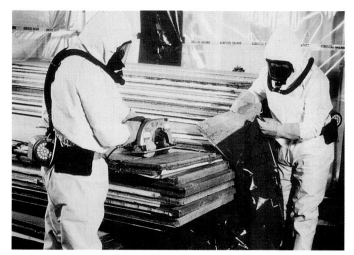

Tyndall beam photography showing asbestos fibres released by mere handling of asbestos boards (left), emphasising the need for proper protection when dealing with asbestos (right).

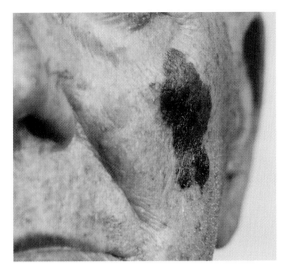

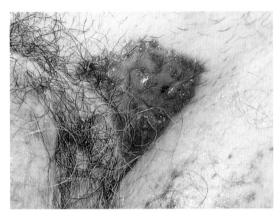

Premalignant melanosis (lentigo maligna) in a man retired after a lifetime of working outdoors.

Epithelioma of groin due to past exposure to mineral oil.

Ultraviolet radiation

Ultraviolet radiation from excessive exposure to sunlight causes both melanotic and non-melanotic skin cancers (basal cell and squamous cell carcinomas).

In Britain few of the 40 000 new cases of skin cancer registered annually are occupationally related. Research shows no consistent increased risk to outdoor workers compared with those of similar socioeconomic status working indoors, but the overall incidence of melanotic skin cancer has almost doubled in 10 years.

Initial presentation may be that of solar keratoses or a premalignant state. Immunosuppression can increase the risk; other possible additive factors are trauma, heat, and chronic irritation or infection.

Mineral oils

The classic epithelioma of the scrotum or groin due to contact with mineral oil is rarely seen today, but these tumours can appear at other sites (such as arms and hands) if contamination with oil persists.

Miscellaneous proved human carcinogens

Agents and exposures	*Target organs*
● Aluminium production	Skin, lung, bladder
● Benzene in petroleum associated industries	Leukaemia
● Bis-(chloromethyl)-ether in production of ion exchange resin	Lung
● Benzene and leather dust in boot and shoe making and repair	Leukaemia, nasal sinuses
● Polycyclic aromatic hydrocarbons and aromatic amines in coal gasification and coke production	Skin, lung, bladder
● Coal tars and pitch in roofing and road maintenance	Skin, lung, bladder
● Ethylene oxide as medical steriliser and chemical intermediary	Leukaemia
● Hardwood dust in furniture and cabinet making	Nasal cavities and paranasal sinuses
● Isopropyl alcohol manufacture	Nasal cavities and paranasal sinuses
● Ionising radiation in nuclear processing, industrial x rays, and medical fields	Various but mainly leukaemia, bone, and skin
● Mineral and shale oils in engineering and metal machining, past exposure to mule spinning in cotton industry and jute processing	Skin, scrotum
● Solvents and pigments in painting and decorating	Various but mainly lung, also oesophagus, stomach, and bladder
● Mists of strong inorganic acid (sulphuric acid) in acid pickling and soap making	Larynx
● Soots from chimney sweeping and flue maintenance	Skin, lung
● Vinyl chloride monomer in PVC production	Liver, brain, lung

Key references
● British Association of Urological Surgeons (BAUS). Occupational bladder cancer: a guide for clinicians. *Br J Urol* 1988;**61**:183–91.
● Duffus JH. *Cancer and workplace chemicals: Handbook No 17.* Leeds: H and H Scientific Consultants, 1995.
● Section 7: Occupational cancer. In: *Hunter's diseases of occupations.* 8th ed. London: Edward Arnold, 1994:623–88.
● Alderson M. *Occupational cancer.* London: Butterworths, 1986.
● *IARC monographs on the evaluation of carcinogenic risks to humans.* Volumes 1–66. Lyons: International Agency for Research on Cancer, 1972–1996.

Other occupational carcinogens

Several other agents are proved human carcinogens. Epidemiological studies now suggest that heavy exposure to crystalline silica dust may increase the risk of subsequent lung cancer. The question of a causal link between electromagnetic fields and cancer, whether in the occupational or domestic context, is still unanswered. Similarly, much recent debate, but finally reassurance, has centred on the potential risk of childhood leukaemia after parental exposure to ionising radiation. Barring accidental exposure, any risk to classified workers exposed to ionising radiation is negligible.

9 BUILDING RELATED ILLNESSES

P H Appleby

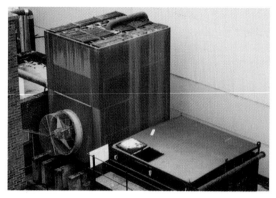

Algal growth on drift eliminators of a building's cooling tower – a potential source of pollutants.

Sick building syndrome

Symptoms associated with sick building syndrome

- Eyes—irritated, itching, dry, watering
- Nose—irritated, itching, runny, dry, blocked
- Throat—sore, constricted, dry mouth
- Head—headache, lethargy, irritability, difficulty in concentrating
- Skin—dryness, itching, irritation, rashes

The idea that buildings can make people ill is one that undermines deep seated beliefs in the function of buildings. Buildings are supposed to provide shelter and a safe environment where people are protected from the elements. The idea of illness associated with manufacturing or mineral extraction is reasonably well understood. However, people becoming ill because of exposure to some unseen agent in their home, school, or office can create a panic out of proportion to the risk.

Building related illnesses fall into two categories: those that have an identifiable cause—such as legionellosis, humidifier fever, and conditions resulting from exposure to known substances such as asbestos, lead in paint, formaldehyde, etc—and those that have no readily identifiable cause but can be described only by a group of symptoms known as sick building syndrome.

The term sick building syndrome is used to describe a situation in a building where more people than normal suffer from various symptoms or feel unwell for no apparent reason. The symptoms tend to increase in severity with the time that people spend in the building and to steadily improve or disappear when people are away from the building.

Symptoms

The symptoms associated with sick building syndrome are those associated with common illnesses and allergies, usually in a relatively mild form so that many sufferers may not see a doctor and may not take time off work.

Risk factors for sick building syndrome

Characteristics of work and building
- Sedentary occupation, clerical work
- More than half of occupants using display screen equipment for more than 5 hours a day
- Maintenance problems identified
- Low ceilings—typically lower than 2.4 m
- Many changes or movements of furniture and equipment
- Public sector tenant or occupant
- Large areas of open shelving and exposed paper

- Sealed building and city centre location
- Large size—typically an occupied floor area greater than 2000 m²
- Centralised control of environmental conditions—no local control of heating, ventilation, etc
- Building more than 15 years old
- Scruffy appearance
- Large areas of soft furnishings, carpets, and fabrics

Environmental factors
- Low room humidities
- Low supply rate of outdoor air
- Smoking permitted in work areas
- Damp areas and mould growth
- Dust, solvents, and ozone emissions from printers and photocopiers
- Low frequency fluorescent lamps creating subliminal flicker

- High room temperatures
- Excessive supply rate of outdoor air
- Dusty atmosphere
- Gaseous emissions (volatile organic compounds) from building materials and cleaning products
- Low frequency noise

Causes

There is no single known cause of sick building syndrome, but there are several risk factors that have been identified from a large number of studies on the epidemiology of the syndrome and investigations of "sick" buildings.

It is evident that some of these factors may combine to cause particular symptoms. For example, eye symptoms may be caused by a combination of long term use of a display screen, low humidity, airborne dust, and irritating airborne solvents.

The increase in use of computers seems to have been a major contributing factor to the onset of sick building syndrome. The additional heat load has led to either overheating or the installation of air conditioning, while the nature of working at a display screen has not only created eye problems but also headaches and musculoskeletal symptoms.

Concern about display screens resulted in a European Commission directive. In Britain this was enacted under the Health and Safety (Display Screen Equipment) Regulations 1992, which requires all users to be trained and provided with certain facilities. From January 1997 all workstations which include a display screen will have to meet the criteria.

Criteria covered by Health and Safety (Display Screen Equipment) Regulations 1992

- Daily work routine of users
- Eye tests
- Provision for training and information
- Risk assessment and analysis of workstations

- Requirements for workstations
  Display screen   Keyboard
  Work desk   Work chair
  Task design   Software
  Environment—heat and noise

Types of building affected

Sick building syndrome not only occurs among office workers. It has been identified in schools, nurseries, libraries, and apartment buildings.

Investigating sick building syndrome

An "outbreak" of sick building syndrome may not be obvious. It may come to light because of complaints to personnel, building maintenance, or occupational health departments rather than to general practitioners.

The Health and Safety Executive have produced the pamphlet *How to deal with sick building syndrome—Guidance for employers, building owners and building managers*. This gives a useful guide to the steps that should be taken before calling in a professional investigator.

Problems with indoor air

Common indoor air pollutants and their sources

Tobacco smoke

Ozone
Source: photocopiers and printers

Volatile organic compounds
Source: Carpets, furniture, building materials, paints, cleaning agents

Dusts
Source: Outdoor air, skin, paper, printer and photocopier toner, mineral and glass fibre

Carbon monoxide
Source: Traffic, combustion (such as gas cookers), tobacco smoking

Oxides of nitrogen
Source: Traffic, combustion (such as gas cookers)

Solvents—Toluene, diphenylmethane, hexamethylene, naphthalene
Typical indoor concentration: 50–10³ μg/m³ (trace outdoors)
Possible sources: Adhesives, sealants, environmental tobacco smoke, wall and floor coverings, paint, moth crystals (naphthalene)

Formaldehyde
Typical indoor concentration: 0–0·6 ppm (0–0·03 ppm outdoors)
Possible sources: Urea formaldehyde foam insulation, fabrics, carpets, floor and wall coverings, adhesives, sealants, lacquer, plywood, chipboard, gypsum board, disinfectants

Concentrations of pollutants in non-industrial buildings are generally orders of magnitude below published limits for occupational exposure. Air quality is rarely a problem in the absence of other factors that contribute to the symptoms which make up sick building syndrome. Exceptions can occur, however, when there are unusual sources of pollution or inadequate ventilation. Larger dust particles in outdoor air should be removed by filters in a building's central air handling plant, which supplies treated air to the building. If these filters are neglected, however, they can become overloaded or disintegrate and provide a source of pollution. If the filters are ineffective, dust will coat the inside of the heating and cooling coils, fans, silencers, and duct work. Where moisture is present, such as in cooling coils that take moisture out of the air, a sludge can form and growth of mould is possible. Dirty air handling systems can also generate odours, which are distributed throughout the building.

Allergies

Airborne allergens in the home

House dust mite excreta
Typical indoor concentration: 0–60 mites/g dust
Possible sources: Carpets, upholstery

Fungal spores—*Penicillium, Cladosporium, Aspergillus, Alternaria, Trichoderma, Stemphylium, Mucor*
Typical indoor concentration: 10–10³ spores/m³ (10⁴ spores/m³ outdoors)
Possible sources: Damp surfaces

Phthalate anhydrides
Possible sources: Epoxy resins

Natural resins
Possible sources: Timber

Insect detritus

Animal proteins

Most airborne allergens (aeroallergens) are organic particles with a mean mass aerodynamic diameter of less than 10 μm. Some are aerosols or vapours.

An allergen's size dictates where it lodges in the airways: smaller particles penetrate the alveoli and cause alveolitis, those of 5–30 μm size tend to lodge in the bronchi and may induce bronchospasm, while larger particles lodge in the nose and give sensitised people rhinitis. Particles that lodge in the eyes may cause conjunctivitis. Allergens of small size, such as some chemicals, may combine with human proteins to cause allergic reactions.

The concentration of allergens in most homes is usually much higher than in offices, particularly in older houses with gardens and pets. House dust mites thrive in mattresses, while moulds grow in gardens, bathrooms, etc.

Action plan to improve air quality in buildings
- Use materials with components of low volatility and low toxicity
- Allow new carpets and soft furnishings to lose most of their volatile component before occupation by workforce
- Minimise use of fibrous materials for finishes and maximise use of wipeable surfaces
- Provide enclosed storage for files, books, and papers
- Ensure there is no penetration by rain or condensation problems
- Ensure that plaster, concrete, etc, has dried out thoroughly before occupation
- Use photocopiers and laser printers with integral devices to reduce ozone production
- Consider banning smoking in work areas
- Isolate dirty and malodorous processes and areas from working or living areas and keep them under negative pressure
- Locate air inlets away from roads and other sources of pollution
- Fit air conditioning and ventilation supplies with high efficiency filters
- Do not allow filters to become too dirty or dirty air to bypass them
- Keep inside of air handling system clean

Exposure to chemicals may be greater in newly decorated and furnished offices, although formaldehyde has been largely phased out by furniture and fabric manufacturers in Britain. The forced movement of air in air conditioned and ventilated buildings may encourage circulation of mould spores and other allergens, especially if they are present within the air handling system itself. Some poorly maintained air handling systems may experience mould growth in filters and humidifiers, although excessive growth is rare.

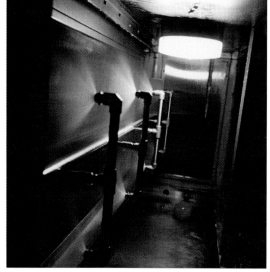

Internal view of spray humidifier in air supply to a building.

Humidifier fever

Actinomycetes are filamentous bacteria which resemble fungi in form and in the types of disease they produce. Thermophilic actinomycetes have been implicated in outbreaks of extrinsic allergic alveolitis such as farmer's lung and mushroom worker's lung, as well as the form of allergic alveolitis called humidifier fever. Not all have an allergic component, and may be due to lung inflammation similar to that caused by organic dust exposure.

A spray humidifier consists of a network of pipes mounted across the airstream. The pipes contain spray nozzles and are connected to a pump which draws water from a tank or pond beneath and through which water is recirculated.

Outbreaks of humidifier fever are rare but generally dramatic when associated with heavily contaminated spray humidifiers or air washers. Occasionally, spray humidifiers have been used to wash out particulates from the air in place of filters. This creates a large volume of sludge which forms in the pond and on downwind surfaces. This sludge can provide the nutrients for microbiological growth.

Legionellosis

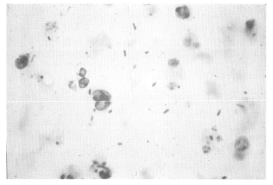

Small, rod shaped bacteria of *Legionella pneumophila* in culture from lung tissue.

Systems and equipment which can be a source of legionellosis
- Evaporative cooling towers and condensers
- Spray humidifiers and nebulisers
- Hot and cold water systems serving taps and showers
- Spa baths and whirlpools
- Horticultural misting systems
- Car washes and lances
- Lathe coolant systems

Legionellosis is a generic term which describes Legionnaires' disease and Pontiac fever. These are relatively uncommon infections, with about 200 cases reported annually in England and Wales, although the reporting rate is thought to be only 10% because the symptoms can be mistaken for other types of pneumonia. These diseases are caused by inhalation of water droplets or particles containing motile thermophilic bacteria of the family Legionellaceae, of which there are some 40 species. The one most commonly associated with Legionnaires' disease is *Legionella pneumophila* serogroup 1, there being 14 serogroups. *L pneumophila* has also been implicated in flu-like illnesses which have been named after the places where they were first reported—that is, Pontiac fever and Lochgoilhead fever.

These bacteria are small and rod shaped and penetrate deep into the alveoli, where they cause infection. There is an incubation period of two to 10 days before the symptoms appear, and it is thought that only 1% of those exposed develop symptoms. The symptoms of Pontiac fever may develop after only five hours or up to three days after exposure.

Although legionella bacteria are found in nature, they tend not to become a problem unless they enter building water systems, which create an aerosol that can be inhaled by susceptible people and which provide a suitable niche for the multiplication of the bacteria.

In its most severe form Legionnaires' disease is a pneumonia that can be fatal or leave the patient debilitated if it is not treated in time. Initial symptoms include high fever, chills, headache, and muscle pain. A dry cough soon develops, and most patients experience difficulty with breathing. Patients may also develop diarrhoea and vomiting and become confused and delirious.

Risk factors in outbreaks of legionellosis

- Water temperature between 20°C and 50°C
- Nutrients available for growth, such as proteins and rust
- Niches which will protect *Legionella* from heat and biocides, such as limescale and sludge
- Fine (invisible) aerosol such as that generated from taps, shower heads, cooling towers, and spray humidifiers
- Low water turnover—temperature may rise, biocides decay, and sediment precipitate to form a sludge
- Open to ingress of animals, insects, dirt, and sun—direct sunlight encourages algal growth
- Susceptible people exposed to aerosol—for example, those with impaired lung capacity or immune system

Recommended further reading

- Health and Safety Executive. *How to deal with SBS–Guidance for employers, building owners and building managers*. London: HMSO, 1995.
- Chartered Institution of Building Services Engineers. *Healthy workplaces*. Balham: CIBSE, 1993. (CIBSE GN2:1993.)
- Health and Safety Executive. *Display screen equipment work*. London: HMSO, 1992.
- Health and Safety Executive. *The prevention and control of legionellosis*. London: HMSO, 1991. (HS(G)70:1993.)

Prevention

Where there is a risk of legionellosis steps should be taken to ensure that equipment and systems are kept as clean as possible and regularly disinfected. If possible, water temperatures should be kept either below 20°C or above 50°C. If this is not possible biocides should be added to the water to prevent legionella bacteria multiplying, provided the biocides cannot enter the indoor air; thus, ongoing treatment of water is not possible with hot and cold water systems or spray humidifiers.

Guidance on the design and maintenance of these systems is given in the Health and Safety Executive's guidance note *The prevention and control of legionellosis*.

10 STRESS AT WORK

Julia von Onciul

Adaptation to the workplace and general adaptation syndrome

Changes in the work environment have led to a change in the balance between physical and mental activity. Technological developments have reduced the amount of heavy physical work. Mental and emotional strain have increased in new working environments that are characterised by lack of time, more uncontrollable factors, background distractions, lack of space, general uncertainty, and more administrative work. The general adaptation syndrome, described by the physiologist Selye in 1975, characterises the process of prolonged exposure to stress and is a useful staged concept.

General adaptation syndrome

1 Alarm reaction
2 Resistance stage
3 Exhaustion stage

Work related stressors

Physical stressors	Emotional and mental stressors
• Noise	• Fear (of sanctions)
• Chemical hazards	• Joy (about promotion)
• Temperature extremes	• Anger (over injustice)
• Physical trauma	• Challenge (of a new position)
• Radiation	• Shock (after sexual harassment or racial
• Poor posture	taunt)
• Vibration	• Competition (with colleague)
• Handling of heavy goods	• Conflicts (with subordinates or managers)
	• Contradictory instructions
	• Negative thoughts
	• Time pressure
	• Structural changes
	• Monotonous tasks
	• Night shifts
	• Overtime

Symptoms of the alarm reaction

- Palpitations—irregular or fast heart beats
- Shallow, fast breathing
- Muscle tension—especially lower back, neck and shoulders
- Dryness of the throat
- Dizziness and lightheadedness
- Numbness of the limbs
- Nausea
- Anxiety
- Sweating

Examples of coping strategies

Perceived psychological stressor: conflict with manager

	Adequate method	Inadequate method
Coping strategy	Talk about issue assertively	Start heavy drinking
Short term effect	Negative—Feeling uncomfortable	Positive—Relaxation
Long term effect	Positive—Self confidence improves	Negative—Secondary problems from alcohol misuse, reduced performance

Perceived physical stressor: constant heavy lifting by geriatric nurse

	Adequate method	Inadequate method
Coping strategy	Plan lifts, use aids	Take time off with bad back
Short term effect	Negative—Taking more time	Positive—Back strain improves
Long term effect	Positive—Less backache, self confidence improves	Negative—Possibility of losing job (too much time off)

What triggers work stress?

Stressors are the agents which trigger the various stress reactions. Today's environment provides physical, emotional, and mental stressors that set off the initial alarm reaction. Physical stressors in factories are usually linked to noise and physical and chemical hazards. Emotional or mental stressors can be unpleasant or pleasant. A promotion can be just as stressful as the loss of a position.

Stressors are additive and can build up. The way in which people are affected depends on their values, experience, and adaptability. A single stressor can become compounded if elements of the established support system fail—for example, if a car breaks down on the way to an important meeting.

1 Alarm reaction

This is the immediate response to a challenge or threat. Mobilisation of the autonomic nervous system triggers the stress response ("fight or flight" response). The various body systems involved coordinate the readiness for action, influencing mood (limbic system), the regulation of the cardiovascular system, breathing, muscle tension, and fine motor activities.

2 Resistance stage

The alarm reaction cannot be maintained indefinitely, and longer exposure to stressors causes people to reach the resistance stage. In this phase people develop a "survival" strategy and a way of fighting against the response the stressor has initiated.

Coping mechanisms may be adequate or inadequate. People tend to prefer short term relief to long term solutions and try to escape uncomfortable situations with a quick remedy. Unfortunately, most easy, short term measures are inadequate because they usually lead to secondary problems such as long term reduction in performance. People need help to identify measures that can lead to long term benefit.

Symptoms of exhaustion stage—Physical disorders

- Tension headaches, migraines
- Irritable bowel syndrome
- Impaired resistence—Colds and other "viral" illnesses
- Potentiation of asthma, dermatitis, psoriasis, backache
- "Gastritis"
- High blood pressure

Symptoms of exhaustion stage—Emotional disorders

- Depression
- Suicidal ideation
- Anxiety syndrome

Symptoms of exhaustion stage—Mental dysfunction

- Accidents or near accidents
- Loss of clarity of thought
- Reduced performance
- Difficulty in concentrating—"Small" but important things are forgotten or mislaid
- Constantly late in spite of enormous efforts to be on time
- Absenteeism
- Increase in mistakes and excuses
- Increase in misunderstandings at work and at home
- Sudden loss of short term memory

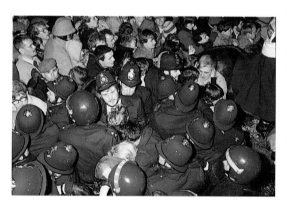

Members of the emergency services are at particular risk of post-traumatic stress disorder.

3 Exhaustion stage

The stress response is healthy in origin and is necessary to keep a person motivated and adaptable. It is when the demands on body and mind are too high or cannot be met in an appropriate way that the person becomes "distressed." Prolonged stress can lead to chronic problems, ultimately an exhaustion of all reserves and energies and even frank depression.

Physical symptoms of impending exhaustion may present with a general feeling of tiredness, lack of energy, and weakness. Non-specific signs can be visual blurring, dizziness, chest tightness, discomfort in breathing, and gastrointestinal symptoms ranging from chronic constipation to diarrhoea and cramps. Sleeping patterns may be disturbed, with difficulty in getting off to sleep and early morning waking accompanied by nightmares. Weight gain or loss is common. Changes in eating patterns range from lack of appetite to overeating or indulging in chocolates. In the workplace people may be able to hide their symptoms unless they become overwhelming, in which case absence from work ensues and the problems present elsewhere (at home or in the doctor's surgery).

Emotional symptoms of stress in the exhaustion stage relate to depression and frustration. These may be manifested in uncontrollable crying; lack of interest in friends, hobbies, and family; and general indifference and reduced attention to personal issues such as exercise, clothes, and eating. In extreme cases self destructive and suicidal tendencies are present. Irritability, coldness, and harshness towards others are often accompanied by extreme guilt. Panic attacks and restlessness can make work difficult and increase stress.

Mental dysfunction in the exhaustion stage presents as a lack of concentration and coordination. This leads to impaired performance and judgment as well as a negative attitude towards work and indecisiveness. In the workplace signs of mental dysfunction are usually noticed more easily than signs of physical illness because they are directly related to performance and thus more apparent to colleagues. The resulting loss of confidence and control disturbs the individual, further reducing performance. Misuse of alcohol, cigarettes, tranquillisers, and other drugs is often observed.

Burnout—This term describes the emotional and psychological results of long continued stress and is based on studies of the social professions, teachers, social workers, and medical staff. Idealistic enthusiasm, conflicting roles, and extreme commitment are typical starting points for the development of this condition, in which mental and emotional exhaustion ultimately lead to apathy and revulsion against everything and everybody.

Post-traumatic stress disorder is a specific form of anxiety disorder following exposure to an extraordinary stressor outside the usual realm of human experience (such as witnessing an armed robbery or fatal accident at work). Subacute or chronic, it is characterised by intrusive psychological re-experiencing of the traumatic event, mental numbness, and symptoms of increased arousal. Emergency services and organisations that experience traumatic incidents (such as intensive care units, banks) often use post-traumatic stress debriefing techniques to prevent development of the disorder. However, their value has not yet been proved. Established post-traumatic stress disorder needs specialised help.

Individual susceptibility to stress

Factors affecting individual susceptibility to stress

- Individual constitution
- Lifestyle and work style
- Coping mechanisms
- Emotional stability
- Previous experiences
- Expectation
- Self confidence

The amount of stress experienced by a person depends on various factors. Heredity plays a role in determining the type of autonomic response and which organ systems will be affected. Other factors are related to lifestyle—such as sleeping and eating habits and behavioural type. The reaction to stress will depend on what strategies are available to the individual—such as relaxation techniques and finding a balance. Work style, organisational skills, attitude towards unpredictable and difficult situations, trust in own abilities, handling of traumatic situations, and "luck" will also determine a person's susceptibility to stress at work.

Factors in the working environment that affect stress

> ## Stressors in the working environment
> - Uncertainty and lack of control (low job discretion)
> - Lack of support from others including coworkers
> - Extreme demands of working environment—long hours, high responsibility, commitment
> - Very low demands leading to boredom, lack of meaning in work
> - Work station—noise, poor lighting, lack of space, extreme temperatures, poor ergonomics
> - Chemical hazards, fumes, passive smoking
> - Organisational culture not allowing for weaknesses—"Are you mental?" "Stress is for wimps"
> - Repetitive tasks
> - Low pay leading to overtime and piecework

Stress is often related directly to the job specifications and working environment or to relationships with people at work, or a combination of both. Conflicts with managers, subordinates, or colleagues may increase as work becomes more pressured. Smaller workforces are expected to do the same or more work, and there is a widespread lack of training in communication and interpersonal skills.

Some of the stress also relates to the identification of a person's role—is the person being asked to be a director or team player? Dissatisfaction is often linked to a lack of autonomy and control in a job.

Dealing with stress

> ## Difficulties in exploring stress at work
> - Patient refuses to relate symptoms to work stress
> - Patient refuses to accept that own behaviour is counterproductive
> - Insufficient information retrievable
> - Other people blamed
> - Non-specific symptoms
> - Long history of illness

> ## Exploring work related stress
> *Ask questions about the following topics*
> - Recent restructuring in working environment
> - Description of workplace
> - Particular worries, especially interpersonal
> - Timing of symptoms in relation to stressors
> - Increase in substance misuse

Doctor's role

The extent of stress at work and its implications are often difficult to investigate and delineate. This is especially so if the symptoms are primarily attributed to a physical condition—for example, headaches ("high blood pressure"), overeating ("obesity in the family"), backache ("scoliosis"). Patients themselves may not want to recognise the presence of stress. For example, those with "type A" personalities often demand a quick, functional, and "easy" remedy for their discomfort, expecting their doctor to miraculously abolish their symptoms.

Information about the working environment may be lacking, either because it is complex—such as a clean room in microchip production—or because of a patient's lack of insight into possible factors in the workplace. It may be difficult to establish whether stress is the result or the cause of a problem at work. Stress may also be part of a wider picture and due to problems outside the working environment—thus, underlying problems in the family or social environment may manifest themselves at work.

If a patient has longstanding stress it may be difficult to trace the origin and trigger of the symptoms. Inquiries about early signs (alarm reaction) can help to identify the start of the problems. With patients who have recently developed symptoms of stress, a few direct questions can indicate a relation to the working environment. Such questioning may help to identify situations that are likely to improve shortly or long term problems that may need closer attention and further investigation.

The root of stress at work may be major changes in the organisation such as new systems of work or problematic colleagues or managers. Impending redundancies, an important deal to close, or an unwanted transfer to a new position can be reasons for worrying. Ask the patient to give a brief description of the work environment—such as factory floor versus office. This may give a clue to the type of stressor encountered—such as noise versus pressure to negotiate a deal. Ask about symptoms occurring typically days before or after a work related stress—a "viral" infection three days after an important meeting, a headache before going to work in the morning or on weekends after a particularly stressful week.

Prescribing drugs—Tranquillisers and β blockers are popular for short term relief of stress but can be disastrous in the long term because of the risks of dependency with tranquillisers and myocardial depression with β blockers. More importantly, they do not treat the root of the problem. For the same reason, antidepressants are not advisable for long term treatment.

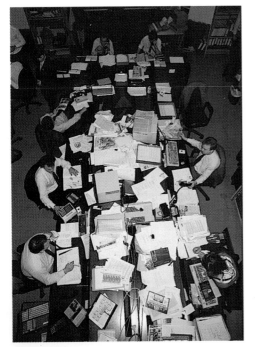

A person's working environment determines what type of stressor he or she may encounter.

Courses that may help to reduce stress at work
- Desk and time management
- Prioritising
- Handling meetings and presentations
- Assertiveness
- Goal setting and problem solving
- Delegating
- Dealing with interpersonal problems

Practical self management for stressed patients
- Take exercise—three 20 minute sessions a week recommended
- Improve posture
- Healthy eating
  Arrange to meet friends to go out for lunch
  Take prepared snacks to work instead of starving all day and overeating in the evening
  Eat and drink less at business lunches and dinners
  Keep soft drinks or water readily available at work
- Stop smoking and drinking alcohol
- Talk to others, such as friends or family
- Listen to tapes and read books
- Take up relaxing hobbies—such as painting but not motor racing

---

Relaxation techniques
- Progressive muscle relaxation (such as Jacobsen technique)—easy to learn, flexible in time (sessions can last 1–30 minutes), can be used almost anywhere and at any time
- Transcendental meditation—develops feelings of refreshment and vitality, 10–15 minutes a day
- Autogenic training—mental circuit training, 10–15 minutes a day
- Alexander technique—reduces lower back pain and tension in shoulder and neck, usually 20 sessions needed to obtain long term benefit
- Martial arts–reduction of tensions through controlled movements (not at work)
- Yoga—fairly complicated technique, experience needed, usually not a short term solution but helpful for some
- Autosuggestion—after initial training applicable to reducing stress before important meetings, etc, but also to reducing addictive behaviour; often needs to be accompanied by other techniques; danger of not treating underlying causes

---

Patient's role

Stress management requires the patient's cooperation and active participation. There are psychological implications, and the patient must take responsibility for his or her actions, thinking about solutions and most probably changing behaviour.

Stress management involves:
- External changes—that is, in lifestyle and working environment
- Internal changes—in behaviour and perception, and in biological response.

Main strategies for reducing work stress include:
- Optimising the workplace where possible and required—get help from an occupational health specialist
- Balancing work stress with a healthy lifestyle and relaxing activities
- Changing personal and work attitude and behaviour where necessary—start with small changes.

Relaxation at work:
- Some techniques are easy to use in a working environment
- Small, frequent breaks (for five minutes every hour) are more relaxing than fewer, longer breaks (for one hour after four hours of continuous work)
- Small physical exercises are useful for computer users
- A few deep breaths with slow exhaling can counteract an immediate stress reaction or panic attack
- Make use of available courses run by psychologists.

Cooperation in managing stress

Multidisciplinary approach to treatment
- Occupational health departments
- Psychotherapy
- Support groups
- Alternative medicine
- Physiotherapy
- Relaxation therapy
- Management training
- Counselling

Further reading
- Makin PE, Lindley PA. *Positive stress management: a practical guide for those who work under pressure.* London: Kogan Page, 1991.
- Chaitow L. *Stress: proven stress-coping strategies for better health.* London: Thorsons, 1995.
- Adams JD. *Stress, health and your lifestyle.* Didcot: Mercury Business Books, 1993.

The photographs of police and stockbrokers were taken by Norman Lomax and Ben Edwards respectively and were reproduced with permission of Impact.

Most workplaces do not employ occupational health staff, but if they do so it is useful to liaise with them as they may be aware of a broader problem affecting several employees and may already be implementing remedial action. There may be an easy solution. An occupational health professional may only take an hour to find out the origin of a problem which resulted in an employee's absence from work.

Counselling—Patients can be advised to attend confidential, non-judgmental counselling over several weeks, in a group or individual setting and usually in one hourly sessions a week depending on need.

Psychological treatment—This should be considered in cases where there is a fundamental psychological issue: for example, a serious lack of interpersonal skills or addictive behaviour.

Other support groups—It is useful to keep a list of bodies and organisations that provide names of support groups, training courses on relaxation, and books on stress management. The last form of support may be a tool for the patient who is unwilling to attend open group discussions.

Recognition—The English courts have recognised that work related stressors can contribute to the breakdown of mental health, reminding employers that they have a duty to ensure their employees' psychological health as well as their physical health. Patients will appreciate it if their doctor recognises that stress is ubiquitous, affecting many people, but allowing of remedial action. It is important to take away the feelings of stigma and failure that often obsess patients with stress symptoms and which lead to an increase in their pressure levels.

11 INVESTIGATING SUSPECTED OCCUPATIONAL ILLNESS AND EVALUATING THE WORKPLACE

Keith Palmer, David Coggon

Conditions that are commonly occupational

- Asthma
- Dermatitis
- Low back pain
- Sensorineural deafness
- Fibrotic lung disease (pneumoconioses)
- Mesothelioma
- Secondary Raynaud's phenomenon

Doctors working in general practice or hospital sometimes encounter patients whom they suspect may have an occupational disease (for example, work related asthma, dermatitis, or fibrotic lung disease). It is important to follow up such suspicions because they may present opportunities for preventing disease or for compensation. Several sources of advice are available, but before others are consulted it is important to obtain the patient's consent, particularly if personal information is to be disclosed. Discussion with the patient is also recommended if any approach is to be made to the employer.

Sources of advice for doctors not working in industry

- Occupational health department at patient's workplace—Many larger employers have their own occupational physicians, who can be approached in confidence
- Health and Safety Executive (HSE)—Telephone number and address of your local regional office should be listed in the telephone directory under "Health and Safety Executive." Inquiries may be directed either to the Employment Medical Advisory Service (medical arm of HSE) or the inspectorate
- Academic departments of occupational medicine—Some centres provide clinics to which doctors can refer patients
- NHS consultant occupational physicians—Growing numbers of NHS trusts employ consultant occupational physicians, who are willing to provide informal advice to colleagues on occupational health problems. A few offer clinics to which patients can be referred

If the patient's employer has an occupational health department the doctor or nurse there can be consulted in confidence. Occupational health staff are bound by the same duties of confidentiality as other health professionals and have special knowledge of the workplace and its hazards. If the company does not have an occupational health service, help can be obtained from the Health and Safety Executive. Their doctors, nurses, and inspectors have a statutory right of entry to all workplaces and respect requests for anonymity (though employers may ultimately suspect the source of a complaint).

Occupational clusters of disease

Apparent clusters are not uncommon in occupational populations and may result from a hazard in the workplace, from shared non-occupational exposures (such as to a hazard in the local environment), or simply from chance coincidence

---

One reason for suspecting that a disease is occupational is the occurrence of a cluster of cases. A cluster of disease is an excess incidence in a defined population, such as a workforce, over a relatively short period. This may range from less than a day for acute complaints such as nausea or diarrhoea to several years for rarer chronic disorders such as cancer.

Apparent clusters are not uncommon in occupational populations. Investigation of occupational clusters sometimes leads to the recognition of new hazards. For example, the link between nickel refining and nasal cancer was first discovered when two cases occurred at the same factory within a year. On the other hand, excessive investigation of random clusters is wasteful of resources. The extent to which an occupational cluster is investigated depends on the level of suspicion of an underlying hazard and the anxiety that it is generating in the workforce. A staged approach is recommended.

Stages in investigating occupational clusters of disease

1 Specify disease and time period of interest. Confirm diagnoses of index cases

2 Search for further cases
Is observed number of cases excessive?

3 What do affected workers have in common? Do their shared exposures carry known or suspected risks?

4 What is known about the causes of the disease?

5 Further investigation
Epidemiology
Clinical investigation

Is there a true cluster?

The first step is to specify the disease and time period of interest and to confirm the diagnoses of the index cases that prompted concern. Sometimes no further action is needed. Of three cases of brain cancer, two might turn out to be secondary tumours from different primary sites. If suspicion remains, it is worth searching for further cases from sources such as data on absence due to sickness. Often, the number of identified cases is clearly excessive, but if there is doubt crude comparison with routinely collected statistics—such as registers of cancers or mortality—should establish whether the cluster really is remarkable.

Manufacturer's information may help in evaluating an occupational cluster—an outbreak of dermatitis among sheet metal workers was found to have occurred because the zinc coating on the metal that they were using had been reformulated, and in combination with a lubricant was producing an irritant effect

Further steps

If an elevated incidence is confirmed the next step is to find out what the affected workers have in common. Do they work in the same job, building, or room, and do they share exposure to the same substances? If so, what is known about the risks associated with shared activities and exposures? This information may come from published reports, but it is also worth checking manufacturers' data sheets and sometimes contacting manufacturers directly about a product. Scientific articles should also be searched to identify known and suspected causes of the disease of interest. Could any of these be responsible for the cluster?

Getting help

At this stage the cause of the cluster may have been identified or suspicions sufficiently allayed to rule out further investigation. If concerns remain it may be necessary to carry out further, more formal epidemiological investigation to assess more precisely the size of the cluster and its relation to work. Help with such studies can often be obtained from academic departments of occupational medicine. Also, patients may need to be referred to specialist centres for investigations such as dermatological patch testing or bronchial challenge.

Evaluating the workplace

Arranging a walk through survey
- Visit by appointment (at least to begin with)
- Check whether you will:
  Be accompanied by someone with respon-
  sibilities for safety
  See someone who can explain the process
  Have a chance to see representative activities
  See documentation on health and safety –
  such as data sheets, risk assessments, safety
  policy, accident book
- Do some preliminary research – identify the
  sorts of hazard likely to be encountered and the
  legal standards that are likely to apply
- If visiting because of an individual's com-
  plaint, discuss it first with the complainant

Assessing the workplace is a major part of investigating occupational diseases. It can provide essential diagnostic clues and is as important as examining a patient. It is also the starting point in preventing injury at work. Once a hazard has been identified, risks can be assessed and appropriate control measures set in place. In addition, by visiting a place of work, the doctor is able to understand better the demands of a job and thus give better advice on fitness for employment.

Normally, workplace inspections are conducted by an occupational health physician or other health and safety professional. However, doctors outside industry may be able to arrange a joint visit by approaching a company's occupational health or safety department. For a doctor asked to advise a company about occupational health, an inspection of the workplace is particularly helpful. Inspections normally take the form of a structured "walk through" survey.

Planning a walk through survey

Industrial processes are often complex, and hazards are plentiful. How should a survey be conducted? The arrangements and context are important. The initial visit should be by appointment (an unan-nounced snap inspection may be more revealing than a planned one, but this is practicable only for a doctor who has an established relationship of trust with the company). The doctor should check the arrangements before visiting: a planned visit saves time, and if no one can be identified who is nominally in charge of safety or if safety data sheets are yellow with age a preliminary diagnosis is already suggested.

The survey should be structured, but the precise way it is organised is less important and at least three approaches are commonly adopted:

Following a process from start to finish—from raw materials in to finished goods out. What hazards occur at each stage? How should they be controlled? Do the controls actually work? This process focused assessment aids basic understanding of the work and its requirements.

A simple hazard checklist
Physical
- Noise or vibration
- Ergonomic
- Radiation or lighting
- Accidents (cuts, falls, burns, fires, explosions etc)
- heat or cold
- Manual handling
- Barotrauma

Chemical
- Dusts
- Fumes
- Gases
- Aerosols and mists
- Fibres
- Liquids
- Vapours

Biological
- Bacteria
- Fungi and moulds
- Insects and mites
- Viruses
- Yeasts

Psychosocial
- Job stress
- Unsocial hours
- Job monotony
- Job organisation

Auditing a single category of activity or hazard (such as dusty or noisy procedures or manual handling) wherever it occurs on company sites. Does the control policy work everywhere, or are there special problems or poor compliance in certain groups of workers or sites? This audit trail or hazard focused assessment is useful for introducing and monitoring new policies (such as a new policy on manual handling).

Detailed inspection site by site—What are the hazards in this particular site? How are they handled? The inspection moves on only when the geographical unit of interest has been thoroughly inspected. This site focused approach is often appreciated by shop stewards and workers' representatives with local ownership of the problem. They may accompany the inspection and often provide insight into working practices and problems not apparent during the visit.

Investigating suspected occupational illness and evaluating the workplace

Simple checklist of control measures

Option	Key questions to ask	Possible controls*
• Avoidance or substitution	Does the material need to be used at all or will less noxious material do job?	Try using a safer material if one exists
• Material modification	Can the physical or chemical nature of the material be altered?	Is it supplied as granule or paste rather than powder? Can it be used wet?
• Process modification	Can equipment, layout, or procedure be adapted to reduce risk?	Can it be enclosed? Can it be extracted? If poured, tipped, or sieved, can the drop height be lowered?
• Work methods	Can safer ways be found to conduct the work? Can it be supervised or monitored? Do workers comply with methods?	Avoid dry sweeping (it creates dust clouds) Be careful with spills Segregate the work; conduct it out of hours
• Personal protective equipment	Have all other options been considered first? Is it adequate for purpose? Will workers wear it?	Provision of mask, visor, respirator, or breathing apparatus suitable for intended use

* A dust hazard is used as an example

What to cover in a walk through survey

Health and safety professionals use checklists to ensure that all the major types of hazard are considered and other checklists to ensure that the various control options are fully explored. They seek to verify that these options have been considered in an orderly and appropriate way:

Firstly, since prevention is better than cure, can the hazard be avoided altogether? Or can a safer alternative be used instead?

Otherwise, can the process or materials be modified to minimise the problem at source? Can the process be enclosed? Or operated remotely?

Have these ideas been weighed before issuing ear defenders and face masks, or other control measures that rely on workers' compliance ("Do not smoke," "Do not chew your fingernails," "Lift as I tell you to")?

A realistic strategy should always place more reliance on control of risk at source than on employees' personal behaviour and discipline.

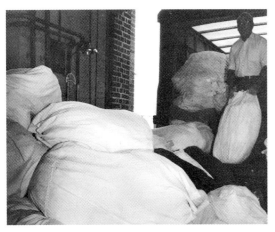

Simple observations can improve safety. In this laundry a shower is provided in case of whole body contamination with bleach, but it is inaccessible.

What the survey may find

The purpose of the walk through survey is to be constructively critical. When good practices and honest endeavour are discovered these should be warmly acknowledged. Faulty practices arise from ignorance as often as from cutting corners. In many small businesses, however, basic errors will be discovered.

We have visited workplaces where expensive equipment, provided to extract noxious fumes from the worker's breathing zone, was switched off because of the draught, or directed over an ashtray to extract cigarette smoke rather than the fumes, or obstructed by bags of components and Christmas decorations.

Exhaust ventilation may be visibly ineffective—the fan may be broken, the tubing disconnected, the direction of air flow across rather than away from the worker's breathing zone; protective gloves may have holes or be internally contaminated; the rubber seals of ear defenders may be perished with age; and so on. There may be no system of audit to check that items of control equipment are maintained and effective. Simple common sense observations, systematically made and systematically recorded, will go a long way towards preventing ill health at work.

Action following the survey

If the evaluation of a workplace is to have a lasting benefit the results must be communicated to senior managers who have the authority to set, fund, and oversee company policies. A written report is advisable, but a verbal presentation, perhaps at a meeting of the company safety committee, may have more impact, as may a small illustrative slide show (see pictures).

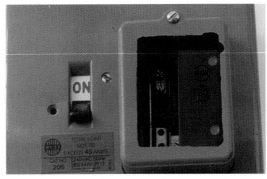

In this fuse box a safety fuse has been replaced with a nail.

The walk through survey may prompt simple improvements or highlight the need for further investigation, such as workplace measurements or a health survey.

Further reading
• Olsen J, Merletti F, Snashall D, Vuylsteek K. *Searching for causes of work-related disease: an introduction to epidemiology at the worksite*. Oxford: Oxford University Press, 1991
• Pittom A. Principles of workplace inspection. In: Howard JK, Tyrer FH, eds. *Textbook of occupational medicine*. Edinburgh: Churchill Livingstone, 1987: 91–106.

12 ABSENCE FROM WORK

Rob B Briner

On one level absence is easy to define and identify: it is simply non-attendance at work by an employee when attendance is expected by the employer. Despite the apparent ease of definition, absence has proved to be a complex phenomenon that resists single or straightforward explanations. The above definition is not, in fact, describing a specific behaviour but rather the non-occurrence of a specific behaviour. In this sense absence is an administrative category rather than a behaviour.

Many different circumstances and behaviours may underlie absence from work. Rather than viewing absence as a single behaviour, making careful distinctions between types of absence is vital for both understanding and managing absence.

> The many types of absence include:
> Absence attributable to sickness
> Voluntary versus involuntary
> Paid versus unpaid
> Distinctions can also be made between:
> Absence events—the number of absence periods of any duration that occur—*and*
> Absence duration

Evidence about absence

> **Costs associated with absence from work**
> ● Lost production
> ● Benefits paid to absentee
> ● Overtime payments for replacement employees
> ● Disruptions to particular sections
> ● Administrative costs of managing absence and rescheduling work

Even quite modest rates of absence can be costly for an organisation. Despite these costs, many organisations maintain surprisingly poor absence records, which means that obtaining good evidence about absence is often difficult. Another difficulty is that, even when organisations keep good records, establishing the types and causes of absence events is problematic.

In many cases it may be impossible to verify employees' claims about the causes of their absence. For example, it is not easy to check whether an employee really had to look after a sick relative or had a migraine or back pain. Questioning employees' claims about absence may also damage employee relations and hence be undesirable from the organisation's point of view.

> **Approximate self reported absence rates due to sickness or injury by occupation and industry***
>
> | Occupation | Absence† | Industry sector | Absence† |
> | --- | --- | --- | --- |
> | Managers and administrators | 3·3% | Other services | 3·5% |
> | Professional | 3·7% | Banking, finance, and insurance | 4·1% |
> | Selling | 4·3% | Distribution, hotels, and restaurants | 4·1% |
> | Associate professional and technical | 4·4% | Construction | 4·3% |
> | Craft and related | 4·6% | Transport and communication | 4·6% |
> | Clerical and secretarial | 4·8% | Manufacturing | 4·7% |
> | Personal and protective services | 5·0% | Public administration, education, and health | 5·2% |
> | Plant and machine operators | 5·4% | | |
>
> * Data from: Office for National Statistics. *Labour force survey.* London: HMSO, Summer 1994, Autumn 1994, Spring 1995.
> † Percentage of employees absent from work for at least a day in previous week

Rates of absence

Although many of the available figures should be treated with caution, some patterns about rates of absence do emerge. First, there are considerable national variations in absence rates. For example, studies in Western Europe have found rates about twice as high as those found in Japan and the United States. Second, there are differences between occupations and sectors of industry in terms of self reported rates of absence due to sickness and injury. There are also differences between categories of disease in the number of self reported annual days off work.

> **Self reported sickness absence by self reported work related illness in Britain***
>
> | Disease | Absence† |
> | --- | --- |
> | Pneumoconiosis | 34 |
> | Hypertension, heart disease, and stroke | 25 |
> | Stress or depression, musculoskeletal conditions, trauma, infections | 20 |
> | Asthma, lower respiratory disease, "RSI," exhaustion, etc | 16 |
> | Hand-arm vibration syndrome, varicose veins, upper respiratory disease, skin disease | 11 |
> | Headache or "eye strain," deafness, eye conditions | 7 |
>
> * Data from: Hodgson *et al* (1993) (see key references).
> † Annual number of days off work per case for each disorder

It should be noted that much of the evidence about absence is self reported and should therefore be treated with caution. However, as indicated above, it is difficult to obtain objective evidence about the causes of absence. Ultimately we may never know the precise causes of an absence event even though employees may be willing to attribute it to a specific cause.

Absence from work

Correlates of absence from work (from several studies)

Corelate	Influence on absence rate
• Increased satisfaction with:	
General job	Slight lowering or no effect
Pay	Slight lowering or no effect
Work itself	Slight lowering
Sense of achievement	Slight lowering or no effect
• Biographical factors	
Older age	Slight lowering or slight raising
Longer tenure	Slight lowering or slight raising
Larger family size	Raising
Sex	Mostly higher in women than in men
• Organisational features	
Larger organisation	Raising
Larger work unit size	Raising
• Job content	
Higher job level	Lowering
More autonomy	Slight lowering or no effect
More responsibility	Slight lowering, slight raising, or no effect
• Other correlates	
Higher commitment	Slight lowering or no effect
Higher job involvement	Slight lowering or no effect
Longer travel distance	Slight raising or no effect

Correlates of absence

Although several correlations have been found, studies have produced very inconsistent results and many correlations are weak. For example, many studies have found no correlation between job satisfaction and absence, while those that have done so found only small negative correlations, indicating that lower levels of satisfaction are only weakly associated with absence. A key point, however, is that correlates of absence have been found with several different factors including attitudes to work, biographical factors, organisational features, and job content.

In most cases, therefore, absence from work is likely to be caused by several factors and any single cause is unlikely to have a strong effect on rates of absence. Some factors, such as age and tenure, have shown both negative and positive associations with absence indicating that these variables may be associated with both higher and lower levels of absence.

Understanding absence

Models of absence from work

Medical model—Suggests that the main cause of absence is injury or sickness

Deviance model—Views employees who are absent as somehow different from other employees: they may have particularly negative attitudes such as laziness and lack of commitment

Withdrawal model—Suggests that employees are absent as a way of withdrawing from unpleasant or unsatisfying working conditions

Economic model—Suggests that leisure and activities outside work are valued by employee; thus, not attending work in order to engage in alternatives is attractive

Cultural model—Identifies causes of absence within social context of organisation and the way shared attitudes and norms influence absence rates: thus, if employees perceive their level of absence to be much lower than that of their coworkers, they may find it easier to decide not to attend work

While sickness clearly can be a cause of absence, many other models are required to build up a comprehensive picture of absence

Several models of absence have been proposed in order to explain it. Given that there are different kinds of absence and different correlates of absence, no single theory is likely to account for all absence events. However, the particular model of absence that is used has implications for the way that absence is managed.

Medical model—Although much absence is attributed by employees to sickness, the available evidence suggests that sickness is not always the true cause. For example, if sickness was a major cause of absence then we would expect absence rates to have fallen over the past 100 years as health care has improved, but rates do not seem to have declined—in fact, they started to rise in all industrialised countries from about 1955. In addition, patterns of self reported diagnosis in relation to sickness absence seem to follow particular trends such as "RSI," "ME," "stress"—indicating that it is the label of sickness rather than sickness itself that may be associated with absence. There is also evidence that receiving a particular diagnosis (such as hypertension) increases absence even where there are no symptoms.

Deviance model—There is some evidence for this model, as a small number of employees often account for a large proportion of total absence in a workforce and one of the best predictors of future absence rates is past absence. While we may be able to identify people who are often absent or absent for long periods, this may be for reasons other than deviance, such as chronic illness or family commitments.

Withdrawal model—This model reflects a common view of absence. However, as indicated earlier, job satisfaction has not been found to be a strong correlate with absence, and evidence for this model is weak.

Economic model—Rather than considering how adverse working conditions may push people away from work, the economic model suggests that employees absent themselves in order to engage in more attractive alternatives. There is some evidence that people who place more value on their time outside work are absent more often. Similarly, when unemployment is high absence rates tend to decrease, indicating that employees may be making some kind of cost-benefit analysis when they decide whether to attend work. If being absent means a greater chance of job loss when jobs are scarce, the relative value of leisure may decrease.

Cultural model—National differences in absence rates support a cultural model of absence, as do figures which indicate that mean absence rates can vary considerably across sites or work units despite other factors that may cause absence being similar.

Managing absence

> Without good information about patterns of absence over time, across work units, and between different types of employee, accurate diagnosis and management of absence is impossible

Techniques for managing absence

Individual techniques
- Negative incentive (punishment)
  Setting expected levels of attendance
  Record keeping
  Investigating absence events (such as interview with superior on return)
- Positive incentive (reward)
  Financial rewards (such as attendance bonuses)
  Other rewards (such as free hours, recognition programmes)

Work techniques
- Job redesign
  Work rotation
  Employee participation
  Physical working conditions
- Influencing attendance
  Establishing group norms
  Flexible working hours
  Company crèche

The basis for managing absence effectively is a comprehensive system of monitoring absence. Now that employers have a greater responsibility for sick pay, many are developing and implementing such systems. Techniques for managing absence may be aimed at individual employees or at changing aspects of the work or the working environment.

Individual techniques include punishments for absence and rewards for attendance. For example, detailed interviews with supervisors on return to work about the causes of the absence can discourage taking time off work. Similarly, issuing warnings and using disciplinary procedures may be disincentives. Disciplinary systems are widely used, yet there is little evidence about their effectiveness. There is, however, evidence that reward systems such as attendance bonus schemes can reduce absence rates.

Changing the nature of the work in terms of job redesign may be effective, but, as indicated earlier, it depends on the extent to which features of the job are actually predictive of absence. Techniques that influence the employees' ability to attend seem to be more successful. The introduction of flexible working hours, in particular, has been shown to reduce absence.

Even with a comprehensive monitoring system, attempts to manage absence are likely to work only if they are approached systematically. In practice implementing a range of measures based on an accurate diagnosis of absence patterns is likely to be most effective. Managing absence also requires a flexible approach to employees who have long term or frequent absences. In some cases specific causes such as chronic sickness or a disability may be identified. In others, however, a range of factors both inside and outside the workplace may be important.

Roles of occupational health departments and general practitioners

Periods of continuing absence attributed to particular illnesses after which employer should seek medical advice*

Illness	Time	Illness	Time
Addiction to drugs or alcohol	6 Months	Mouth and throat disorders	1 Month
Anaemia (except in pregnancy)	4 Months	No abnormality detected	Immediate
		Nervous illnesses	3 Months
Arthritis (unspecified)	6 Months	Postnatal conditions	6 Months
Back and spinal disorders	6 Months	Respiratory illnesses:	
Concussion	1 Month	Asthma	6 Months
Fractures of legs	6 Months	Upper respiratory tract	
Fractures of arms	2 Months	infection	1 Month
Gastroenteritis, gastritis,		Bronchitis	2 Months
diarrhoea and vomiting	1 Month	Skin conditions, dermatitis	
Haemorrhage	3 Months	eczema	2 Months
Headache	1 Month	Sprains, strains, bruises	1 Month
Hernia (strangulated)	6 Months	Ulcers:	
Inflammation and swelling	1 Month	Perforated	9 Months
Joint disorders except		Peptic	2 Months
arthritis	3 Months	Varicose	6 Months
kidney and bladder		Corneal	2 Months
disorders	3 Months	Cuts, abrasions, burns,	
Menstrual disorders,		blisters, foreign body	1 Month
dilatation and curettage	3 Months		
Miscellaneous, anorexia, fainting, giddiness, insomnia, investigation, undiagnosed, obesity, observation, tachycardia	1 Month		

* Times suggested by Department of Social Security (from *Statutory Sick Pay Manual*, CA30, published by the Contributions Agency of the DSS). Employers are entitled to set their own time thresholds, above which they start inquiries.

Occupational health departments and general practitioners play important roles in managing absence attributable to sickness. In the past 10 years changes in legislation have altered these roles.

When statutory sickness certificates were required from the first day of absence, general practitioners were inundated with patients with minor illnesses that they felt were sufficiently serious to keep them away from work. People with high rates of sickness absence therefore made considerable demands on their general practitioner.

Self certification has ameliorated this unsatisfactory situation but has moved the responsibility for deciding the seriousness of short term sickness from patient and doctor to employee and employer. As noted earlier, questioning employees about their claims of sickness may be resented and can be difficult and embarrassing for employers.

Some employees may believe they have to take time off for particular conditions. For example, an employee with a minor cold may not attend work for fear of infecting colleagues, or a person with back pain may believe that he or she must remain in bed. Clearly, doctors have a role in providing basic health education and clarifying the advisability of attending work. In some cases—such as food handlers who have diarrhoea—the doctor may have to advise someone who may feel both willing and able to work to stay away.

Role of occupational health department or general practitioner in managing sickness absence

- To confirm that employee is sufficiently ill to warrant absence
- To assess likely pattern of absence associated with that illness
- To assess whether employee's previous pattern of sickness absence is likely to be repeated
- To confirm that employee has an ongoing medical problem but that amount of sick leave is greater than would be expected. A medical review can be suggested at this point
- To separate domestic causes from sickness and possibly to give opinion on whether there are work related causes
- The review can be presented in non-medical terminology and in such a way as to preserve doctor-patient confidentiality

Typical procedure for employer dealing with repeated short term absences

- Counsel the employee
- Investigate the causes of absence thoroughly and openly
- If absence is result of an accident at work complete an accident report form, and if absence is for more than three days also complete a RIDDOR form
- Seek medical advice through occupational health department, which will obtain employee's permission to approach his or her treating doctor. Or contact the treating doctor directly, with employee's permission under Access to Medical Reports Act 1988
- When there is an underlying cause for absence consider possible solutions—other duties, transfer to another department, light work, flexible working arrangements, retirement on grounds of ill health
- If spells of sickness are intermittent but too frequent and other solutions fail, caution the employee
- When there is no underlying cause counsel the employee that disciplinary action will result if there is no improvement in absence
- Set a time limit to review the situation for any improvement
- If there is no improvement start disciplinary procedure, leading to a final warning and dismissal on grounds of incapacity

Employers clearly wish to reduce absence, including absence attributable to sickness, and an occupational health department can help employers manage sickness absence more effectively, in a way that may be fairer and that preserves medical confidentiality. Whether rates of sickness absence can be reduced clearly depends on several factors such as its present level (it may already be very low) and the specific illnesses encountered. As discussed above, however, accurate absence records are a vital first step in managing any type of absence.

Sickness absence that will certainly lead to permanent incapacity to do a particular job may be dealt with by medical retirement if such a scheme exists. The most difficult situation is when there is chronic sickness of an intermittent type, such as asthma, but permanent disability is not anticipated.

Another problem is when sickness absence is partly caused by the employee's own actions, such as alcohol misuse. Sickness may also combine with other factors, at work or at home, to causes absence. It may therefore be helpful to look at some cases of sickness absence in a wider context in order to improve management.

Not all employees (or employers) realise that a person can be legitimately dismissed for unacceptably high rates of absence attributed to sickness (whether "genuine" or not) provided that a proper management procedure is followed (see box opposite).

Absence from work: final comment

Key references
- Fitzgibbons DE. A critical examination of employee absence: the impact of relational contracting, the negotiated order, and the employment relationship. *Research in Personnel and Human Resources Management* 1992; **10**: 73–120
- Hodgson JT, Jones JR, Elliot RC, Osman J. *Self-reported work-related illness: results from a trailer questionnaire on the 1990 labour force survey in England and Wales.* HSE Books, 1993.
- Huczynski AA, Fitzpatrick MJ. *Managing employee absence for a competitive edge.* London: Pitman, 1989.
- Johns G. Understanding and managing absence from work. In Dolan SL, Schuler RS, eds. *Canadian readings in personnel and human resource management.* St Paul, MN: West, 1987: 324–35.

People are inclined to use their own preferred or pet theories to explain whatever absence they happen to observe. Interestingly, the theories that people use to explain their own absence are often different from those they use to explain the absence of others. Thus, we may feel that our own absence is legitimate and necessary yet regard the absence of others, particularly if it is regular or prolonged, with suspicion. However, a key point to remember is that taking a single approach when considering and managing absence is unlikely to be successful. Absence is not a single or simple phenomenon and should not be treated as such.

13 ASSESSING FITNESS FOR WORK

William Davies

Assessments of fitness for work can be important for job applicants, employees, and employers. Unfitness due to an acute illness is normally self evident and uncontentious, but assessing other cases may not be straightforward and can have serious financial and legal implications for those involved. Commercial viability, efficiency, and legal responsibilities lie behind the fitness standards required by employers, and it may be legitimate to discriminate against people with medical conditions on these grounds. Unnecessary discrimination, however, is counterproductive if suitable staff are overlooked and may be costly in cases of unfair dismissal. In addition, the Disability Discrimination Act 1995 makes it illegal for employers of 20 or more staff to discriminate without justification against those with disability as defined by the Act.

Fortunately, balancing these often complex socioeconomic and legal issues to achieve a sustainable decision on fitness is not primarily a medical responsibility. Doctors do, however, have responsibilities to assess the relevant facts competently and provide helpful medical advice when required.

Sociolegal implications of assessing fitness for work
- Security of employment
- Rejection at recruitment
- Occupational ill health or injury
- Justifiable or unfair discrimination
- Retirement due to ill health
- Termination of contract
- Claim for unfair dismissal
- Industrial tribunal
- Medical appeals
- Litigation for personal injury
- Criminal prosecution
- Professional liability

Basic principles and responsibilities

Key concepts of health and safety

Hazard
The potential of a thing, condition, or situation to cause harm

Risk
The probability of harm occurring from a hazard

Negligible risk
The most widely held view of negligible risk in the context of health and safety is an annual risk of less than one in a million

Competent assessment
A competent assessment requires a level of detail, consultation, and consensus broadly commensurate with the nature of identifiable hazards and the extent of reasonably foreseeable risks

Staying on track

This chapter deals with assessing fitness for "identified employment." To avoid confusion with related issues, the following points should be noted at the outset:
- Fitness for work in relation to retirement benefits for ill health will depend on the specific provisions of the pension scheme, and general guidance is available[1]
- The recently introduced "**all work** test" of fitness is not related to identified employment but concerns entitlement to social benefit (incapacity benefit) and is the responsibility of the Benefits Agency Medical Services' doctors[2]
- The Disability Discrimination Act 1995 does not in principle change good medical practice in assessing fitness for work but obliges employers to be more accommodating to those covered by the legislation
- Key concepts of health and safety, risk assessment, and risk management—hazard, risk, negligible risk, and competence—apply to assessing fitness for work and should be clearly understood.

Medical responsibilities

General and hospital practitioners

To patient
- Act in patient's best health interests

To Department of Social Security
- Apply the "**own occupation** test"*
- Complete forms med3, med4, etc, when required

- Supply on request relevant clinical information

*The test is whether the person by reason of some specific disease or bodily or mental disablement is incapable of work which that person could be reasonably expected to do in the course of their occupation

Detailed advice on the above is available in the guide IB204[2] and from regional Benefits Agency Medical Services Centres

Occupational health practitioners

To patient
- Act in patient's best health interests

To employer
- Assess functional ability and occupational risks
- Make recommendations on fitness in accordance with valid predetermined standards
- Provide information and advice that enables management to make an informed decision on compatibility of subject with employer's requirements and legal responsibilities

Detailed advice on the above is available in *Fitness for Work. The Medical Aspects*[1] or from accredited specialists in occupational medicine

Medical responsibilities

Doctors' responsibilities vary according to their role. General practitioners and hospital doctors have direct responsibilities to the patient and also obligations to the Department of Social Security associated with applying the "**own occupation** test." Occupational health practitioners have direct responsibilities to the employee or job applicant and the employer.

These groups may take different approaches but have important common ground. If patients, employees, and job applicants are to be treated fairly every medical opinion on their fitness for a job should be based on a competent assessment of relevant factors and should satisfy the same basic criteria. Patients' interests will be best served when there is, between doctors, clear understanding, due consultation, and, as far as possible, agreement.

Key principles of assessing fitness for work

1 The primary purpose of the medical assessment of fitness to work is to ensure that the subject is fit to perform the task required effectively and without risk to the subject's or others' health and safety

2 The subject's fitness should be interpreted in functional terms and in the context of the job requirements

3 Employers have a duty to ensure, so far as is reasonably practicable, the health, safety, and welfare of all their employees

4 Legal duties of reasonable adjustment and nondiscrimination in employment are imposed by the Disability Discrimination Act 1995

5 Good employment practice involves due consideration of the needs of all job applicants and employees with disabilities or medical conditions

6 It is ultimately the employer's responsibility to set the objectives for attendance and performance and to ensure compliance with the law on health and safety and employment

Reporting the outcome as a medical recommendation—or, when appropriate, as medical conclusions and medical advice—should enable management to make an informed decision on the compatibility of the subject with the employer's requirements and responsibilities

Key principles in practice

The first principle establishes three basic criteria for fitness—attendance and performance, health and safety risk to others, and health and safety risk to self. In this context "without risk" reflects a fundamental ethical concept of occupational medicine which limits medical discretion: doctors should not presume to decide for others that risks are acceptable; employers must take this responsibility and require medical advice on the nature and extent of risk to make informed decisions.

The second principle means that an appraisal of the subject's medical condition and functional ability—that is, a medical-functional appraisal—together with a review of the relevant occupational considerations should provide an empirical assessment of ability and risk. This assessment may be judged against the required fitness criteria to determine what the outcome should be.

The third, fourth, and fifth principles point to the potential there may be for preventing or controlling risk and for accommodating the needs of people with disabilities or medical conditions. Such measures are effectively enabling options, which, if available, may justify a conditional recommendation of fitness.

The sixth principle means that technically all decisions on fitness rest with the employer. This is because the employer determines what is required of the employment and ultimately carries responsibility for the risks.

Outcome

When fitness criteria are defined and the assessment clearly satisfies or fails to satisfy the employer's requirements and responsibilities, a "medical recommendation" of fitness can be made (see green columns in desktop aid at end of chapter). When fitness criteria are uncertain—when the employer's requirements and responsibilities cannot be predetermined or presumed—the "medical conclusions" of the assessment should be made clear to the employer. In addition, a medical view on the potential for enabling options or on the appropriateness of employment or continued employment may be given as "medical advice" (red columns in desktop aid).

Assessment of ability and risk

Medical-functional appraisal

History and examination
- Pre-employment questionnaire or health declaration
- Health interview – occupationally relevant direct questions
- Physical examination focusing on job requirements

Work related tests and investigations
- Perceptual – Snellen's, Ishihara's, City University, voice tests, audiometry
- Functional – spirometry, peak flow, strength tests
- Physical endurance and aerobic capacity – step test, bicycle ergometer
- Diagnostic (health on work) – exercise electrocardiography, drug and alcohol tests
- Diagnostic (work on health) – haematology, biochemistry, urine analysis, radiographs
- Functionally specific questionnaires – respiratory (MRC), pre-audiometry

Consultation and research
- Details from general practitioner and medical specialist
- Details from other specialists – such as psychologist, audiologist
- Advice or second opinion from specialist occupational physician
- Advice or second opinion from independent specialist – such as cardiologist, neurologist
- Review of texts, journals, and research

Data sources for standards of fitness

- Key publications[1 3 4] – For drivers, pilots, food handlers, and many other occupations
- Health and Safety Executive[5-7]
- Government departments – For teachers[8]
- Professional associations – ALAMA (Association of Local Authority Medical Advisors) for firefighters, police, teachers, etc, and ANHOPS (Association of National Health Occupational Physicians) for health care professions

Medical-functional appraisal

Doctors should always have a basic knowledge of the job demands and working environment before undertaking a medical-functional appraisal so that the extent and emphasis of the appraisal may be tailored accordingly. Any medical conditions that could pose a risk to the subject's or others' health and safety or that could affect attendance and performance should be identified and evaluated.

A suitably constructed questionnaire is the simplest form of assessment, and, for pre-employment screening, a questionnaire or health declaration will be sufficient to permit medical clearance in many categories of employment.

Some occupations have statutory standards, and appraisals must include measuring necessary factors. Others have standards set by authoritative recommendations or guidance. If no guidance exists doctors must judge how extensive the assessment should be by taking account of the nature of any medical conditions identified, the type of work, and the reasons for management's request for medical advice.

Occupational considerations

In straightforward cases a medical-functional appraisal and the doctor's existing knowledge of the job demands and working environment may be sufficient for a recommendation of fitness. However, a closer look at occupational factors is often needed to determine the precise requirements of the job, the subject's real abilities in a working environment, the nature of any hazards, and the probability of harm occurring (the actual risk in the workplace).

- A subject may be able to show satisfactory ability in a job simulation exercise despite a physical impairment that might have affected fitness – for example, a work related test of manual dexterity for an assembly line worker with some functional loss due to a hand injury
- In teaching, health care, and many other occupations perceived hazards of epilepsy are often found to be negligible when the potential for harm to others is properly assessed
- If diabetes is well controlled the risk of injury from hypoglycaemia may be found to be very remote when the true frequency and duration of hazardous situations are taken into account.

Enabling options

A subject's potential fitness often depends on intervention. There may be unexplored treatments that can be provided. Rehabilitative support may be needed to achieve or speed recovery. Employers can make reasonable adjustments, temporary or permanent, to meet the needs of people with medical conditions. Prevention and control measures can reduce or eliminate health and safety risks that would otherwise prohibit a recommendation of fitness.

- Unexplored treatments that are often identified during assessments include physiotherapy, anxiety management, psychotherapy, and hormone replacement therapy
- A tailored, stepwise rehabilitative programme can make the prospect of returning to work after serious illness less daunting and may be vital for recovery from anxiety, depression, occupational stress, and other demotivating conditions
- Modifying a job specification may allow a recommendation of fitness with minimal inconvenience to the employer—for example, removing the requirement to undertake occasional lifting for an arthritic subject
- Substituting a sensitising or irritant product may, with other sensible precautions, enable an asthmatic or eczematous employee to continue working as, say, a paint sprayer or cleaner.

These measures may be applicable under the Health and Safety at Work Act. The Disability Discrimination Act 1995 may also require reasonable adjustments to be made. Even if intervention is not obligatory, employers may recognise the benefits of positive action. Doctors should therefore always bear these options in mind as it may be possible to give a conditional recommendation of fitness that the employer would be willing to accommodate.

Fitness criteria in difficult cases

The above approach should produce a reliable opinion in most cases, but further steps may be needed if the parameters of the fitness criteria are uncertain. In a fitness assessment this may occur with one, two, or all three of the criteria. Dealing with the issues in turn is advisable.

Attendance and peformance

The possible impact of a medical condition on a subject's ability to meet required levels of attendance and performance is a major source of employers' requests for medical opinion. The doctor's responsibility is to give the most accurate opinion that the circumstances allow. Conclusions and advice should be as positive as possible without misrepresenting the facts and discussed with the subject. This should help motivation and may improve recovery.

● Open ended statements such as "Unfit; review in three months" are not welcomed by employers, who prefer uncertainties to be expressed as probabilities—"Mr Smith has been incapacitated but is progressing well and is likely to become fit to return to work within four weeks."

● If social or motivational factors are evident discuss these with the subject, and advise management accordingly—"Mrs Jones' incapacitation is due to family commitments that are likely to continue for the foreseeable future. She realises that her employment could be at risk and would welcome an opportunity to discuss her situation with management."

● It may be necessary to ask management for an appraisal of capabilities before making definitive conclusions on the relevance of medical factors—"I will therefore require a management report on her progress after week 6 of the rehabilitation programme."

● In cases of prolonged sickness absence, do not be pressured into recommending ill health retirement for doubtful reasons—"Mr Green is likely to remain unfit for the foreseeable future, but there are not sufficient grounds for ill health retirement under the pensions scheme."

Health and safety risk to others

Employers have a legal duty to ensure the health and safety of employees and the public. In principle the doctor identifies hazards and quantifies any risks while management decides on a subject's fitness based on the medical conclusions and advice. In practice, however, doctors confirm fitness when there is no risk and unfitness if there are clearly unacceptable risks. For the many cases that lie in between, there may be confusion as to whether it is a management or medical responsibility to decide on fitness. A pragmatic approach is suggested:

● For negligible risk, the doctor may advise that the subject be considered fit provided that the judgment of negligible risk is made objectively and based on a competent assessment and that the employer applies all reasonably practicable precautions

● For greater than negligible risk, the doctor should define the type of hazard and extent of risk as clearly as possible to enable management to make an informed decision.

Advice from a specialist occupational physician may be required to confirm the competence of the risk assessment or to assist management on acceptability.

Health and safety risk to self

The principles of assessing risk to others apply here, but medical advice can go further. In some cases employment may pose a risk of ill health, but the employer is satisfied that everything possible has been done to prevent or reduce risks—for example, the risk of relapse in a teacher with a history of work related anxiety—depressive disorder.

To advise that in such cases the subject should always be deemed unfit because of a risk of work related ill health is unrealistic. The benefits of employment for the subject, and possibly the employer, may considerably outweigh the risks. On the other hand, there could be issues of liability for both employer and doctor if the risks are overlooked.

The autonomy of the subject must be reconciled with the needs and responsibilities of the employer. Legal precedent does not provide clear guidance on how this should be done; the issues are complex and the implications serious. A rational basis for providing helpful medical advice involves a full discussion of the prognosis with the subject to determine where the balance of benefits and risks lies.

● If the subject thinks the benefits outweigh the risks and the doctor agrees, advice should be given in support of employment, providing the assessment and the judgment of balance between benefit and risk have been competently undertaken

● If the subject thinks the benefits outweigh the risks but the doctor cannot agree, seeking a second opinion from a specialist occupational physician should be considered before providing management with definitive advice

● If the subject thinks the risks outweigh the benefits and the doctor agrees, early retirement should be considered

● If the subject thinks the risks outweigh the benefits when the hazard and risk seem disproportionately low then motivational factors (such as a common law claim or ill health retirement incentives) may be relevant. If so, the doctor should proceed cautiously and consider obtaining a second opinion from a specialist occupational physician.

The conclusions should be presented to management in context, indicating the nature of hazard, the extent of risk, and strength of medical consensus. This will enable the employer to discharge his or her responsibility in a complex area with the benefit of such medical support as the circumstances allow.

Definitive opinion

The conclusions, recommendations, and advice outlined above are valid only for the specific fitness criterion addressed. In each case the outcomes of all three criteria should be consolidated to provide an all embracing definitive report. The desktop aid (overleaf) includes a synopsis of the outcomes commonly encountered and may be adapted as a classification guide for audit purposes.

Desktop aid – Framework for assessing fitness for work

Assessment of ability and risk		Fitness criteria		Outcome
• Medical-functional appraisal • Occupational considerations • Enabling options	+	• Attendance and performance • Health and safety risk to others • Health and safety risk to self	=	• Conclusions • Recommendations • Advice

Applying fitness criteria – Synopsis of outcomes

Attendance and performance

A Subject's condition compatible with required levels of attendance and performance	B Attendance or performance limitations due to medical conditions or disabilities identified but likely to resolve	C Attendance or performance limitations due to medical conditions or disabilities identified and likely to remain for foreseeable future	D Subject's performance and capabilities cannot be determined by medical assessment alone	E Subject's conditions clearly incompatible with requirements of post and likely to remain so
	(a) in forseeable future because of anticipated recovery or (b) if certain enabling options can be accommodated (such as treatment, rehabilitation, reasonable adjustments, or risk prevention)	Do not overlook social or motivational factors which may be relevant. Discuss implications with subject. If necessary seek advice*	Feedback on performance is required to identify possible impact of medical conditions	Help subject come to terms with implications such as ill health retirement, termination of contract, redeployment (if available), or rejection (at pre-employment stage)
Recommend fit	*Advise of conclusions indicating (a) likely timescale and/or (b) relevance of enabling options Review as necessary*	*Advise of conclusions Review as necessary*	*Advise of medical issues as far as possible and of need for management appraisal Review as necessary*	*Recommend likely to remain unfit*

Health and safety risk to others

F No risk to others	G Risk identified but preventable	H Negligible risk	I Risk greater than negligible but may be acceptable	J Risk to others clearly unacceptable and likely to remain so
	Identify and pursue relevant enabling options such as treatment, rehabilitation, reasonable adjustment, or risk prevention	Ensure judgment of negligible risk is made objectively and based on competent assessment (if unsure seek advice*) and that management applies all reasonably practicable precautions	Inform management of nature and extent of risk as clearly as possible. Specialist occupational physician may be able to help management in deciding on acceptability*	Help subject come to terms with implications such as ill health retirement, termination of contract, redeployment (if available), or rejection (at pre-employment stage)
Recommend fit	*Advise fit (subject to specified conditions)*	*Advise fit (subject to specified conditions) Review if circumstances change*	*Advise risk cannot be dismissed as negligible and that acceptability is for management to consider*	*Recommend likely to remain unfit*

Health and safety risk to self

K No risk to self	L Risk identified but preventable	M Risk identified which subject thinks are outweighed by benefits	N Risks identified which subject thinks outweigh benefits	O Risk to self clearly unacceptable and likely to remain so
	Identify and pursue relevant enabling options such as treatment, rehabilitation, reasonable adjustment, or risk prevention	*If doctor agrees* - Ensure assessment and judgement of balance between risk and benefit have been competently undertaken (if unsure seek advice*) *If doctor disagrees* - consider obtaining second opinion before advising	*If doctor agrees* - Consider early retirement *If doctor disagrees* - If risks seem disproportionately low consider relevance of motivational factors (such as common law claim or ill health retirement incentives) If present proceed cautiously and consider obtaining second opinion*	Help subject come to terms with implications such as ill health retirement, termination of contract, redeployment (if available), or rejection (at pre-employment stage)
Recommend fit	*Advise fit (subject to specified conditions)*	*Advise of conclusions in context*	*Advise of conclusions in context*	*Recommend likely to remain unfit*

Definitive opinion

The conclusions, recommendations, and advice outlined above are valid only for the specific fitness criterion addressed.
In each case the outcomes of all three criteria should be consolidated to provide an all embracing definitive report.

*Advice and second opinions should be obtained from doctors with training and expertise to provide proper assistance.
Specialist accreditation/certification for occupational physicians (MFOM, FFOM) is awarded via the Royal College of Physicians Faculty of Occupational Medicine.

1   Cox RAF, Edwards FC, McCallum RI. *Fitness for work. The medical aspects.* 2nd ed. Oxford: Oxford Medical Publications, 1995.
2   Benefits Agency, Department of Social Security. *A guide for registered medical practitioners (IB204). Medical evidence for statutory sick pay, statutory maternity pay, and social security incapacity benefit purposes.* London: DSS, 1995.
3   Medical Advisory Branch, DVLA. *At a glance guide to current medical standards of fitness to drive.* Swansea: DVLA, 1996 March.
4   Taylor JF. *Medical aspects of fitness to drive, a guide for medical practitioners.* 5th ed. London: Medical Commission on Accident Prevention, 1995.
5   Health and Safety Executive. Your patients and their work, an introduction to occupational health for family doctors. Bootle: HSE, 1992.
6   Health and Safety Executive. *Pre-employment screening.* London: HMSO, 1982. (Guidance note MS20.)
7   Health and Safety Executive. *Health aspects of job placement and rehabilitation—Advice to employers.* London: HMSO, 1989. (Guidance note MS23.)
8   Department for education. *The physical and mental fitness to teach of teachers and of entrants to initial teacher training.* London: DE, 1993. (Circular No 13/93.)

14 WORKING WITH AN OCCUPATIONAL HEALTH DEPARTMENT

Anil Adisesh, Gordon Parker

> ## Aims of an occupational health service
> The promotion and maintenance of the highest degree of physical, mental, and social wellbeing of workers in all occupations
>
> World Health Organization 1950

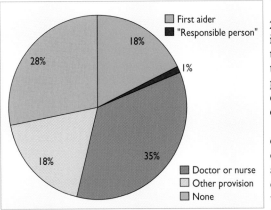

Provision of occupational health facilities for all employees in United Kingdom (adapted from Bunt 1993).

First aider
"Responsible person"
18%
1%
28%
18%
35%
Doctor or nurse
Other provision
None

One in 14 consultations with a family doctor by patients of working age is for a condition that is due to work or that affects ability to work. General practitioners are often in the best position to make an early diagnosis of occupational illness, to prevent further problems by taking appropriate action, and to facilitate a return to work after illness or injury. Hospital specialists also need to consider the possibility of work related causes for an illness and the effects of the illness and treatment on future fitness for work. Therefore, doctors in both primary and secondary health care should be aware of the role and responsibilities of occupational health services and work with them for patients' benefit.

Occupational health services are not distributed uniformly among the 24 million people employed in the United Kingdom; their provision is influenced by the size of the company and the nature of the industry. In the public sector (NHS, civil service, etc) 72% of employees have access to a doctor at the workplace compared with only 20% of workers in the private sector. There is no statutory responsibility in Britain—in contrast to other European countries—for employers to provide an occupational health service or even access to an occupational physician.

Many large employers in the private sector (and increasing numbers of NHS trusts) have occupational health services headed by a specialist occupational physician and supported by occupational health nurses and ancillary staff. Smaller firms may have services headed by an occupational health nurse. Medical communication may therefore be with a specialist occupational physician, a local general practitioner or other doctor providing advice on a part time basis, or a nurse. Some doctors may find it unusual to communicate with a nurse practitioner, but the ethical considerations remain the same.

Occupational disease

> ### Case history of an occupational disease
> A 42 year old hospital cleaner presented to the occupational health department of an NHS trust with hand eczema. He had been referred by his manager, who was concerned about his fitness to continue his domestic cleaning duties. He had seen his general practitioner but had not improved much despite using topical corticosteroids and emollients over a three month period.
>
> His work involved stripping varnish from floors. He mentioned that some of the chemicals he had to apply were caustic, and he wore rubber gauntlets when diluting them. Occasionally, he had got some on his hands, which caused skin irritation for a few days. After stripping the floor, he had to spray on a wax solution and then polish the floor with the machine. The occupational health physician obtained a list of all the chemicals used and the manufacturers' materials safety data sheets. There were several chemical irritants such as ammonia. There were preservative agents in the wax solution, and at least one, ethylenediamine, was a known sensitising agent.
>
> A letter was written to the patient's general practitioner suggesting that the eczema might have an occupational cause and that a dermatology opinion would be useful. The general practitioner arranged a referral, and, after patch testing, contact allergic dermatitis due to ethylenediamine was diagnosed. The occupational health department reviewed the work practices of the man's job and recommended improvements. An alternative wax without the sensitising agent was identified, and a substitution made. The patient's rash resolved.

Doctors should always be alert to the possibility of a disorder having an occupational origin and should take a patient's occupational history if appropriate. If occupational disease is suspected the first point of contact for advice should be the employee's occupational health service. The occupational health team will have a wealth of experience and will know about the hazards in the workplace and their potential effects, and they will readily pass that information to doctors caring for an employee.

A single case may be a "sentinel" that could allow identification of others or protection of colleagues also at risk. Occupational health departments may initiate or be prepared to take part in relevant research projects when new problems are recognised or further evaluation of known hazards is useful.

If there is no occupational health service at a patient's workplace the Employment Medical Advisory Service, based in the regional Health and Safety Executive office, can give advice and will investigate working conditions and hazards when necessary. Local NHS consultants in occupational medicine will readily offer general advice and may be able to accept referrals for specialist opinion.

Communication

Reasons for requests for information by occupational health services

- Pre-employment—to aid in assessing fitness for a particular job
- During sickness absence—to provide details about diagnosis and prognosis
- During resettlement or rehabilitation—to aid return to work and give all available assistance
- Ill health retirement—to support an application, when a return to work is not feasible

Example of a doctor's letter to a manager that is unclear and contains too many medical terms

Dear Harry,

Mr A was in good health until 1989, when he suffered a coronary thrombosis. He made a good recovery until about 1993, when he began to complain of constant ache in his legs that worsened on exercise. He has now got persistent ache in both legs and an exercise limitation of about 200 yards.

He recently had an episode of hemianopia affecting the right eye, in which the outside half of the vision in this eye disappears. This is due to vascular disease of the eye and is related to his generalised vascular disease indicated by his coronary thrombosis and by his leg pains. He also complains of the recent onset of some shortness of breath, and when I examined him I found that his heart beat was irregular.

Mr A has quite severe generalised vascular disease, and his life expectancy is not good. However, the only problem affecting his ability to work at the present time is his difficulty in focusing, the result of his recent eye problem. This should, with luck, improve sufficiently for him to be able to undertake his work in the office. Provided no further disaster occurs, he should be able to resume employment in 3–4weeks. However, as I said previously, his prognosis is extremely poor. I hope this is of some help to you.

Yours sincerely,

Example letters

1 Request for information from occupational health department

Dear Dr

Your patient Ms B works as a secretary for this company. Her managers have referred her to me because of the excessive amount of sickness she has had over the past two years (about 60 days a year), and they are concerned that she may continue in this vein. When I saw her recently she told me that she suffers from anorexia nervosa, for which she is being treated with antidepressants and counselling.

I would be most grateful if you could let me know any significant facts about her medical history, her current treatment, and any thoughts you have on the likely prognosis. With this information, I will be able to advise her managers as to her likely working capacity and perhaps suggest some job modification if that would be helpful. I enclose her written permission for me to approach you on this subject under the Access to Medical Reports Act and would like to thank you in anticipation of a quick reply.

Yours sincerely,

2 Unhelpful reply from general practitioner

Dear Dr

Thank you for your letter about Ms B. I am sorry for the delay in replying. I have seen Ms B recently. In my opinion she had good results from the treatment, and I think she is quite fit to continue her employment as a normal person. Please send a cheque for £50 as a fee for this report.

Yours sincerely,

3 Helpful reply from general practitioner

Dear Dr

I have known Ms B for three years and last saw her for review on 8/8/96. She has had anorexia nervosa since the age of 15. For the past month she has been treated with fluoxetine 40 mg daily. Her response to this increased dose has been encouraging, with her weight now at 42 kg. She will begin a course of psychotherapy in four weeks' time on an outpatient basis. I plan to review her progress in three months.

Ms B will probably have a lifelong tendency to an eating disorder. However, with early intervention at any indication of relapse, I am confident that her lifestyle and work should not be greatly affected. I will continue to review her at three monthly intervals over the next year, but I would be happy to see her sooner if this became necessary. I enclose an invoice for my fee for this report.

Yours sincerely,

Communication between a patient's employer and his or her doctor is usually initiated by the occupational health service requesting medical information. It is in everyone's interest to get patients back to work as safely and quickly as possible and to prevent their premature return. This requires rapid and accurate communications, but the greatest delays occur when the treating doctor fails to answer a request for information—though to be fair, the Access to Medical Reports Act is sometimes to blame because it gives patients 21 days to signify if they wish to see a report before it can be sent. Delays often cause problems for patients and possibly financial loss if they cannot work or perform overtime while awaiting a decision on fitness for work.

Occasionally, a request for information may come directly from a manager or personnel department. Such requests should also be accompanied by the employee's consent under the Access to Medical Reports Act. In this situation it is important to establish whether the report will go to a doctor retained by the company or to a lay person (manager). A lay person may not fully understand a report containing medical jargon, which could be misinterpreted or give rise to unnecessary concern to the detriment of the patient. Reports received by an occupational health department, however, will be held in medical confidence, and medical terminology may aid understanding. The implications for work can then be explained to management with advice based on knowledge of the work environment.

Medical information

When doctors are asked for medical information it is important that their report is comprehensive. In the example shown, if Ms B is in danger of losing her job because of her excessive sickness absence, the first report does not give the occupational physician much basis to dissuade management from this course of action.

The second reply confirms the diagnosis, describes current treatment and response, gives plans for further treatment and follow up, and provides a prognosis. With this information, and after discussion with Ms B, the occupational physician can say that she is receiving suitable treatment for her condition, that arrangements for follow up are in place, that management should allow her time for regular hospital visits, and that, subject to regular review by the occupational health department, she is not likely to have much greater sickness absence than her colleagues.

Such information is useful to employers, who generally do not want to "fire and hire" staff as there are considerable costs associated, human as well as economic, and greatly prefer to retain trained staff. Invoices for fees should be enclosed or attached and must not contain confidential information as they may have to be passed to finance departments for payment.

Example of a letter from a consultant physician to support a patient's application for a job*

Dear Sir/Madam

I am writing in support of Ms C's application to work abroad as a field worker in a remote tropical location.

In 1995 Ms C had a right leg deep vein thrombosis, which was treated with warfarin, but one month later she had a pulmonary embolus. Eight months after this, in January, she had an acute illness with fever and a vasculitic rash. A diagnosis of systemic lupus erythematosus was made, and she was treated with prednisolone. In June she had an epileptiform seizure due to cerebral lupus. Glomerulonephritis was diagnosed on renal biopsy in July; the changes were consistent with lupus. She was treated with azathioprine in addition to prednisolone. She then developed hypertension.

The current situation is that she has heavy proteinuria indicating active glomerulonephritis, but she seems clinically well. Her treatment is prednisolone 10 mg daily, azathioprine 100 mg daily, bendrofluazide 5 mg daily, propranolol 320 mg daily, and prazosin 10 mg twice daily. She will need to continue taking immunosuppressants for the foreseeable future, but her short term outlook is good, although her renal function is likely to deteriorate in the longer term. Given her fortitude with illness, I am sure she would make an excellent field worker for the project.

Yours sincerely,

*The medical facilities available, or the lack of them, and the risks of disease in an immunosuppressed person have not been considered

Doctor's opinions

The treating doctor's opinions about fitness to work may be unhelpful when these have not been specifically asked for, particularly if the patient is aware of the opinion. For example, a general practitioner may consider that a "process worker" who is being investigated for syncope is fit to be at work: however, the safety of the patient and others in the workplace may be at risk if the doctor is not aware of the patient's duties—such as working alone in a control room, wearing breathing apparatus, etc.

Conversely, the treating doctor may consider another patient, for example, a nursing care assistant, to be unfit to return to work after a resolving back strain because her job involves heavy lifting. After assessing the care assistant, the occupational physician may advise management that she can return to work provided that she undertakes no manual handling of patients or of loads greater than 10 kg. This may still allow a wide range of useful work to be undertaken, and it is the skill of management to accommodate such advice. A telephone conversation between the treating doctor and the occupational health department may help clarify the options available in managing a return to work.

In the rare event of complete disagreement between an occupational physician and a general practitioner or specialist on a patient's fitness for work, industrial tribunals tend to follow the occupational physician's opinion. They regard the occupational physician as being in fuller possession of all the facts, both clinical and relating to the actual work to be done, and thus in a better position to make a balanced and independent judgment.

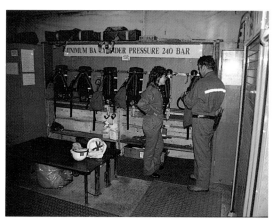

High standards of medical fitness may be required for some aspects of work—such as using breathing apparatus.

Ethics and confidentiality

Some doctors are wary of releasing medical details to occupational health professionals, believing that medical confidentiality may be compromised and information given to the employer. This should never happen. All communication between occupational health services and other doctors is held in strict medical confidence.

Communication by occupational health services to managers is generally made in broad terms without revealing specific medical details. From a medical report indicating that an employee has angina on exertion, the occupational physician may inform management: "Mr D has a medical condition which prevents him from working in the loading bay and performing other heavy manual work. He should be fit for his other duties as a senior storeman and will be kept under regular review." It is not necessary for management to be aware of specific medical details, but, for some conditions (such as epilepsy), it may be helpful for work colleagues to be told of the problem, with the patient's agreement, so that appropriate help can be given (or unhelpful actions avoided).

Some doctors may also believe that occupational health services usually act in the interests of the employer rather than in those of the employee or patient. To behave in this way would be contrary to the ethics of occupational health practice, but this misconception still inhibits useful communication. In fact the occupational health service acts as an independent and objective advisor to the individual and to the organisation, hopefully to their mutual benefit.

- All requests for information from general practitioners or hospital specialists are governed by the Access to Medical Reports Act (1988)

- Written consent is needed for the occupational health physician or nurse to contact the treating doctor, and the consent form should be attached to the request

- The patient has the right to view any report before it is sent to the occupational health service to correct factual errors, to ask the doctor to amend the report, to add their own comments, or to refuse to allow the report to be sent. After all, it may contain information which the patient might consider prejudicial and therefore needs to be fair and accurately expressed

Other communications with occupational health services

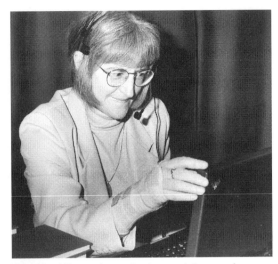

Valuable skills can be retained at work by use of appropriate aids – such as a voice recognition dictation system linked to a laptop computer for an employee no longer able to type rapidly. (Reproduced with subject's permission.)

Further reading

● Health and Safety Executive. *Your patients and their work, an introduction to occupational health for family doctors.* Suffolk: HSE Books, 1993.
● *Guidance on ethics for occupational health physicians.* 3rd ed. London: Faculty of Occupational Medicine Royal College of Physicians, 1993.
● Cox RAF, Edwards FC, McCallum RI. *Fitness for work, the medical aspects.* 2nd ed. Oxford: Oxford University Publications, 1995.
● Bunt K. *Occupational health provision at work.* Suffolk: HSE Books, 1993. (HSE Contract Research Report No 57.)

The photograph of a computer with voice recognition system was produced by Mr D Griffiths.

Health promotion and health screening

Health promotion and general health screening—such as for coronary risk factors—may be practised in the workplace in accordance with the Health of the Nation initiatives. There is potential for duplication of effort and confusion if general practitioners are unaware of such programmes. Occupational health services are responsible for informing general practitioners of their reasons for undertaking any investigations and for informing employees and their medical advisers of any abnormal findings. Occupational health services can get a bad reputation by undertaking health screening in a disorganised or unprofessional way and leaving general practitioners to pick up the pieces.

Rehabilitation and resettlement

Facilities such as physiotherapy, counselling, and access to "fast track" or private health care may be available through the workplace. For employees who become disabled or for new employees with a disability, the local placing, assessment, and counselling team (PACT) may be usefully involved. Patients may benefit from the early use of such services and, as a result, may recover and return to work sooner. The occupational health department will be able to advise management in specific terms about suitable work to facilitate an employee's return to work rather than simply advocating "light duties." Liaison between the medical services helps to optimise this process.

Ill health retirement

Sometimes medical conditions preclude a return to work, because of permanent incapacity for a particular job, and information will often be requested in order to support ill health retirement. Alternatively, it may be necessary to explain why an employee's job is to be terminated due to incapacity (when a person has not attended work for an excessive period because of sickness absence, but recovery of fitness is envisaged), which is a managerial decision. The pension fund's grounds for ill health retirement may be explicit and leave little room for clinical opinion or may be quite open.

There is potential for disagreement between the occupational physician and other medical advisers, particularly if restricted duties or redeployment are viable propositions. Although these options are becoming infrequently available in the current economic climate, it is preferable that views are discussed openly and an equitable decision made. If work has been a causal factor in the illness then civil litigation may arise against the employer. The interface between occupational health departments and other health services care providers should therefore be open and two way, initiated by either party whenever discussion of patient care in relation to employment could be advantageous.

15 WOMEN AT WORK

Laila H Kapadia

More and more women seek paid employment outside the home, and, by the year 2000, they will make up 45% of the Western world's workforce. Almost half work part time. Women, whether working or not, still generally bear the greater share of housework, child care, and care of elderly people.

Reductions in sexual discrimination and the influence of the women's liberation movement now allow women to enter almost any occupation, however physically demanding or apparently unsuitable. In some countries, mainly developing ones, women are the mainstay of the agricultural working population. In others, such as those of the former Soviet Union, women predominate in medicine and engineering. Equal opportunities legislation in socially developed countries outlaws sexual discrimination and ensures job retention during and after pregnancy, allowing women to continue working throughout their reproductive span. Despite all this, in all societies women's work is less prestigious and less well paid.

Although women live longer than men (84 v 79 years in Britain) and are more interested in their health, they suffer greater morbidity, take more drugs, consult their general practitioners more often, are more frequently admitted to hospital, and take more time off work (though the reasons for this are not as clear as they may seem—see chapter 12).

Medical advances for women at work

Contraception has allowed women to space their pregnancies but has also resulted in their postponing pregnancy to a later age (possibly to avoid interrupting their careers), increasing the risk of obstetric complications

Advances in medicine, not least a more holistic approach by gynaecologists, have helped women by controlling symptoms that were once common reasons for absence from work—dysmenorrhoea, menorrhagia, and perimenopausal symptoms. Intrauterine surgery, outpatient investigations, and day case treatments can expedite a return to work. On the other hand, fertility treatment can, because of its inflexible timing, mean periods away from work and can be attended by the side effects of drugs and tension and anxiety that may affect performance at work.

Specific conditions

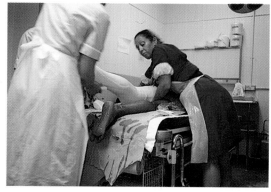

Lifting patients by hand—a traditional practice that is being phased out.

Postnatal depression occcurs in 10% of women to varying degrees and may persist for a year or longer in about a third of the most severe cases

Backache

Women share men's high rate of work related back pain. In terms of occupation, a greater burden falls on the health services because of the large amount of manual handling in a predominantly female workforce. Women probably get backache to the same degree as men who work in heavy, awkward, or repetitive jobs. Backache is rarely gynaecological in origin. It is, however, common in pregnancy and after the menopause due to osteoporosis.

Psychiatric and psychological morbidity

Childbirth is associated with substantial psychiatric morbidity, most of it occurring in women who were previously well. Mood disorders occur more often after childbirth. Termination of pregnancy for fetal abnormality can be traumatic, but psychological effects may be greater when termination is unrelated to fetal wellbeing. In the latter case work colleagues are less likely to know why a woman is showing signs of grief.

Women are particularly at risk from sexual discrimination in occupations that are traditionally male dominated, such as the armed forces, police, medicine, and the highly competitive world of top executives and the money markets

Menopausal symptoms that can affect performance at work

- Hot flushes and night sweats
- Emotional and sexual problems
- Urinary frequency and urgency
- Musculoskeletal weakness

Cancers in women

Cancer	No of cases/year	
	New cases	Deaths
Cervical	4 500	2 000
Ovarian	5 000	4 500
Breast	27 000	16 000
Lung	12 000	10 000

Health of the Nation's targets for reducing ill health and death

1 Coronary heart disease and stroke
2 Cancers—lung, breast, cervical, skin
3 Mental illness
4 HIV and AIDS and sexual health
5 Accidents

Screening can prevent 50–70% of cervical cancers. The incidence of cervical cancer is increasing in 20–34 year olds and decreasing in 40–50 year olds. However, mortality from cervical cancer is falling, probably due to screening

Management of menstrual disorders

- Certain conditions such as polycystic ovaries should be considered, and anorexia nervosa sometimes presents as amenorrhoea
- Most menstrual irregularities are now dealt with in general practice and can be treated with hormones, antiprostaglandins, or antifibrinolytic drugs
- The value of dilatation and curettage has been questioned
- Hysterectomy for older women suffering from menorrhagia is no longer the automatic solution offered by gynaecologists—hormonal manipulation or endometrial ablation may be more appropriate
- Outpatient specialist investigation for menstrual problems by ultrasound imaging and laparoscopic diagnosis (with the possibility of minimally invasive surgery) have revolutionised diagnosis

Other specific anxieties that may cause poor performance at work or absence are false positive results from screening during pregnancy, the trials of assisted reproduction, premenstrual syndrome, and psychological symptoms around the time of the menopause. Difficulty in making decisions and loss of confidence may be features of the menopause itself.

Women undoubtedly suffer from discrimination in jobs that are traditionally male dominated. All kinds of discriminatory and excluding behaviour have been described, from treating women as unequal colleagues or merely decorative to frank verbal or physical sexual harassment. It is hardly surprising that this may result in anxiety and loss of confidence.

Menopause

The average age of the menopause in Britain is 50. There are about 10 million postmenopausal women in the United Kingdom, many of them still at work. Those who worked part time when their children were growing up may return to full time work at this age.

Menopausal symptoms may affect the working day. Hot flushes can be very embarrassing at work, and night sweats may lead to insomnia and daytime tiredness. There may also be emotional and sexual problems that can cause anxiety but do not relate to work directly, although they may make work related psychological problems harder to bear. Urinary symptoms of frequency and urgency may be a problem for women working long shifts or without easy access to toilets. Musculoskeletal weakness and ligamentous laxity may predispose to aches and pains which can affect any lifting or handling. Premature menopause, especially if it is iatrogenic, is more likely to give severe symptoms and require hormone replacement therapy.

Pelvic pain

This may cause short term absence from work. It may be acute, presenting as cramps and low central abdominal pain just before the start of menstruation in young women and is sometimes accompanied by nausea, diarrhoea, and flushes. After the age of 30, painful periods tend to be associated with pelvic disease such as pelvic inflammatory disease or endometriosis.

Chronic pelvic pain, defined as lasting longer than six months and with no abnormality at laparoscopy, may arise from structures of the abdominal wall or disease of the gastrointestinal or urogenital tract or skeleton. This is more likely to reduce performance at work.

Cancers

Cancers in working women may cause anxiety, morbidity, and mortality. As the workforce gets older, there will be more working women with cancer. The government's Health of the Nation targets breast, cervical, and lung cancer. The workplace is an ideal venue for education and health promotion. A no smoking policy at work may help people to give up, healthy food can be provided in workplace canteens, and breast and cervical screening can be promoted by allowing reasonable time off work to attend.

Menstrual disorders

Heavy menstrual bleeding is experienced by one in three women at some stage in their lives, and periods of amenorrhoea may also occur. Young women who move to a new job in another part of the country often miss periods initially. Counselling at work can often help women anxious about menstrual irregularity.

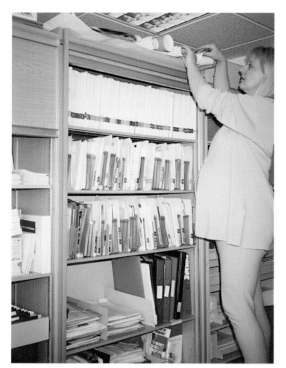

A pregnant woman may have difficulty fulfilling all her usual duties, and these may need to be temporarily adjusted.

Pregnancy

New legislation was introduced into the Management of Health and Safety at Work Regulations 1992 with effect from 1 December 1994 to implement the European Directive on Pregnant Workers. This puts a duty of care on employers to provide a safe system of work to all women of reproductive age, their unborn children, and all working mothers who are breastfeeding. It also introduced protection against loss of income, establishing a woman's right to return to her job and to have the time spent in antenatal care remunerated. The Workplace (Health, Safety, and Welfare) Regulations 1992 recommend that facilities be provided for pregnant women and nursing mothers to rest (ideally, including facilities for lying down) and be conveniently situated in relation to sanitary facilities.

The statutory minimum maternity leave is now 14 weeks (regardless of length of service and how much money is paid out), six weeks of which is paid at 90% of full time salary. Statutory maternity pay is given for 18 weeks, which must be continuous, and the woman is protected against dismissal for ill health during this period and has full rights with regard to pensions, holidays, etc, in addition to any existing contractual rights. Some employers improve on this, especially for long serving workers.

Laws on health and safety already cover most of these areas, as a safe workplace is where both men's and women's health is taken into account. If a risk is identified during pregnancy, and risks must by law be identified and assessed in the spirit of the COSHH regulations, the employer should
- Temporarily adjust the woman's conditions or hours *or*
- Move the woman to another job *or*
- Give the woman paid leave.

Doctors may be asked to supply a certificate stating that a pregnant employee should be moved from night work on grounds of health and safety. Doctors (or midwives) may be asked for a certificate to confirm pregnancy for an employer earlier than the Maternity B form.

Hazards at work

Assessment of risk at work during pregnancy

Employers are required to carry out a formal risk assessment wherever it is thought that elements within work might pose a risk to pregnancy

Physical hazards
- Handling
- Repetitive tasks (carpal tunnel syndrome is potentiated)
- Vibration
- Extremes of temperature
- Ionising radiation
- Work posture
- Travelling
- Tendency to fatigue

Chemical hazards
- Solvent, rayon, dyes, and viscose in the chemical, pharmaceutical, plastics, rubber and textile industries
- Herbicides, insecticides, and fungicides used in farming and market gardening
- Heavy metals—especially lead, chromium, and mercury
- Ethylene oxide used for disinfection

Biological hazards
- Abortion or stillbirth can be caused by *Listeria* or parvoviruses
- Congenital abnormalities may be caused by rubella
- Acute infection with certain viruses such as herpesvirus may cause intrauterine death
- Transmission of infection at birth with HIV or hepatitis B

There are potential hazards to women of childbearing age from the handling of specific chemicals and more general physical hazards. The effects may be direct or indirect and are varied, ranging from effects on libido, fertility, and menstruation to miscarriage, premature labour, and the outcome of pregnancy. Fertility and fecundability can also be affected via male partners' exposure to work related hazards.

Computer display screens—Some women's greatest worry is still that of exposure to computer display screens during pregnancy, and there are still instances of women being excluded quite unnecessarily from working with screens because of a perceived risk of miscarriage or fetal malformation. There is good evidence that such exposure causes neither of these effects. For women who are pregnant and who work at a display screen, there may be ergonomic issues that should be taken into account, and the office working environment should be assessed.

Hazardous chemicals—Certain industries are known to present particular hazards to pregnant women, and there is a large body of literature about the effects of exposure to specific chemicals that can cause miscarriage or birth defects. Remember that chemicals, especially when combined with solvents, can be absorbed through the skin (such as hormones developed for pharmaceutical purposes), and by inhalation. Some substances that are handled are teratogenic or mutagenic (such as cytotoxic drugs). The effects of chemicals on the fetus are difficult to disentangle from those caused by smoking, misuse of alcohol or drugs, inadequate antenatal care, poor nutrition, and poverty. Generally, the risks are highest in early pregnancy, so advice should be given to women who are planning pregnancy as well as those already pregnant.

Infections—About 3% of newborn infants have important congenital malformations, but infections contribute to only about 5% of these. All such infections are by no means associated with work, but at least those acquired from preparing food, working in laboratories, and handling animals are preventable.

Women at work

Further reading

● Health and Safety Executive. *New and expectant mothers at work – a guide for employers* Bootle: HSE, 1994.
● *European directive on pregnant workers – Management of health and safety at work regulations 1992.* (ST No 2051.)
    Amended in 1994 (ST No 2865).
● Schnorr TM, Grajewski BA, Hornung RW, Thun MJ, Egelund GM, Murray WE, *et al.* Video display terminals and the risk of spontaneous abortion. *N Engl J Med* 1991;**324**:727–33
● McDonald A. Work and pregnancy. In McDonald JC, ed. *Epidemiology of work related disorders*. London: BMJ Publishing, 1995:293–323.

The photograph of nurses lifting a patient was taken by Tom Webster and is reproduced with permission of Impact Photos.

Working during pregnancy

There is such variation in pregnancy that no hard and fast rules can be given. A healthy, problem free pregnancy will have hardly any impact on work but might make women who are having a difficult pregnancy feel guilty that they cannot keep up at work. There are many non-specific problems to consider such as fatigue (which occurs more rapidly in pregnancy), backache, nausea and vomiting, and a change in the body's centre of gravity. Mental concentration may be affected by the metabolic changes of pregnancy.

Thus it is important to consider all aspects of a woman's work as soon as she becomes pregnant to see if modifications would help. These may include adjusting the number of hours worked, the nature of the work done, increasing rest periods, substituting daytime working for night work, being flexible about working hours, or providing varied work to prevent problems associated with a static posture. Physical demands should not be excessive, especially in late pregnancy. If it is considered unsafe on medical grounds for a pregnant or breastfeeding woman to be working at night, she must be transferred to daytime work or, if this is not possible, given paid leave.

In general work has been shown to have a beneficial effect on pregnancy, and most studies show no adverse outcomes in healthy women with a normal pregnancy.

16 LEGAL ASPECTS

Martyn J F Davidson

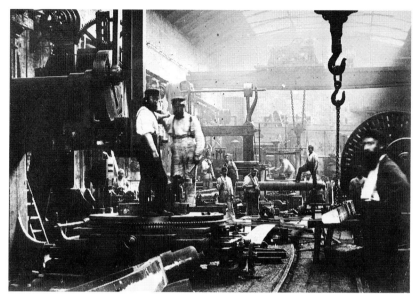

Extremely hazardous conditions in 19th century factories led to development of health and safety legislation.

People do not expect their work to damage their health. Employers have a legal and a moral duty to safeguard the health of their employees. The legal framework defining this duty was established in the 19th century. Though prompted by humanitarian concerns, these legal developments were the pragmatic result of the concerns of industry—the supply of healthy workers required to increase productivity was threatened by the toll of premature death and disability. Duties on employers to safeguard the health and safety of their workforce have gradually developed from both statute and common law.

Reporting of occupational diseases

<table>
<tr><td colspan="2">

Comparison of reporting systems

RIDDOR
- Established in 1986
- Participants—British employers
- Reporting rates estimated at 44% by the labour force survey (injuries only); only 10% among self employed
- Total of 504 cases (all reportable diseases) in 1994–5
- Most common reported diseases:
  Hand-arm vibration syndrome 305 cases
  Occupational asthma 74 cases

SWORD
- Established in 1989
- Participants—British consultant chest physicians and occupational physicians
- Participation rates 72%
- Total of 3305 cases reported in 1994
- Most common reported diseases:
  Asthma 968 cases (29%)
  Mesothelioma 643 cases (19%)
  Benign pleural disease 735 cases (22%)

EPI-DERM
- Established in 1993
- Participants—British consultant dermatologists and occupational physicians
- Participation rates 67%
- Total of 3449 cases reported in May 1994 to April 1995
- Most common reported diseases:
  Contact dermatitis 2722 cases (79%) (especially related to nickel and to rubber/thiuram, particularly among female cases)

</td></tr>
</table>

RIDDOR

Current levels of work related illness are difficult to ascertain accurately. Employers are required by statute to report cases of occupational disease under the Reporting of Injuries, Diseases and Dangerous Occurrences Regulations 1995 (RIDDOR)—recently updated with effect from 1 April 1996, with modest changes from the 1985 original. The list of reportable diseases has now been brought into line with the list of prescribed diseases. Previously, only 28 conditions were listed, with many important omissions such as occupational dermatitis. An employer needs to report a case of occupational illness only after being notified of the diagnosis by a doctor.

Data for RIDDOR are underreported for several reasons. Employers have no incentive to report, since to do so will often trigger a visit from the enforcement authority. Neither the patient nor the treating doctor may realise that a condition is work related, and they may be unaware of the need to inform the employer of the diagnosis.

The Health and Safety Commission, which collates and publishes these figures annually, commissioned a labour force survey in 1990. This survey estimated that only a third of reportable illness is actually reported and that 2·2 million cases of work related illness had occurred in the preceding year. A further survey is in progress, with broader data collection, and is to be published in 1997.

Voluntary reporting

Good data are vital if the extent of occupational disease is to be recognised and a strategy formed for prevention. Two successful voluntary schemes are the SWORD (surveillance of work related and occupational respiratory disease) and EPI-DERM (occupational skin disease) projects. Their data suggest a much higher burden of disease than other sources. From 1 January 1996 these schemes are combined within OPRA (occupational physicians reporting activity), which is also intended to collect data on musculoskeletal injuries, hearing loss, and any other serious illness, particularly neurological or psychological.

Compensation

There are essentially two systems with the potential to compensate an employee with occupational illness: the prescribed disease scheme or the civil courts. Success in one does not guarantee success in the other.

Prescribed diseases

Several well recognised occupational diseases are "prescribed" for benefit by the Department of Social Security under the industrial injuries scheme. Thirty nine prescribed diseases are listed in the Social Security (Industrial Injuries) (Prescribed Diseases) Regulations 1985. They fall into four categories, each denoted by a capital letter—those that are due to physical (A), biological (B), or chemical (C) agents or those of a miscellaneous nature (D).

The Industrial Injuries Advisory Committee advises on the addition of new prescribed diseases. Its criteria for prescription have traditionally been narrow—the disease must be a recognised risk to workers in a particular occupation and not a risk to the population in general. Also, the causal link between disease and exposure must be well established. Compensation depends on the degree of disability, as assessed by the local adjudication officer from the Department of Social Security. Medical evidence is submitted by an adjudicating medical authority, or special medical board in the case of respiratory disease. There are also separate arrangements for occupational deafness. The numbers of cases assessed under the scheme give further data on these diseases.

Civil claims

Civil law has developed to compensate one person for damage received through another's action or inaction. Most civil claims will be brought under the tort, or civil wrong, of negligence. That is, the employee will argue that the employer failed in his or her duty of care to safeguard the worker's health. In a civil court the plaintiff (employee) must show (*a*) that the defendant (employer) owed the worker a duty of care, (*b*) that the employer negligently breached that duty, and (*c*) that the employee suffered damage as a result of that breach.

The depth and breadth of the duty of care has been developed over the years by landmark cases. The concept of the "reasonable and prudent employer, taking positive thought for the safety of his workers in the light of what he knows or ought to know" was clarified by Judge Swanwick in 1968. Exactly when an employer should be aware of a health risk in the workplace is inevitably contentious, particularly in relation to claims for occupational illness. Courts will often decide on a "date of knowledge," after which no employer could reasonably claim ignorance. This date will often relate to government guidance or other influential advice.

Large damages may seem impressive when reported in the media, but the adversarial system as presently practised is not an entirely appropriate way of dealing with such cases. Some would argue that it is neither fair nor equitable. Furthermore, if state compensation has been paid for an industrial disease before the civil claim, this may be clawed back from awarded damages in excess of £2500. The Compensation Recovery Unit, established in 1990 for this purpose, had reclaimed a total of £281m by February 1995.

Lord Woolf, in his recent proposals for reform, has suggested a fast track system to speed up small claims. Alternatives such as the no fault compensation systems practised in other countries may have some advantages, but these have not found favour in Britain.

The expense of bringing an action, plus the liability for costs if unsuccessful, excludes many claimants who do not qualify for legal aid (and the criteria for qualification seem to be ever more limiting). From July 1995, solicitors have been able to enter into conditional fee agreements for certain classes of proceedings. If the plaintiff is unsuccessful the solicitor goes unpaid. If the plaintiff wins, the solicitor is paid a success fee, or uplift, in addition to the standard fee. The plaintiff may also insure against the cost of losing an action. These changes may open up litigation to claimants who would not previously have been able to take the financial risk.

Criminal Law

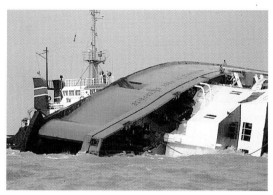

The Zeebrugge ferry disaster resulted in a failed manslaughter charge.

Criminal law offers other sanctions to protect the health and safety of employees, though these avenues do not provide compensation for individuals. British criminal law arises from statute: acts of parliament, and regulations made thereunder, provide the "rules" by which employers are expected to abide. Case law, courts' decisions in specific cases, provides guidance on the interpretation of these rules. The judiciary also develops the common law by this means. Decisions made in higher courts are binding on lower courts.

The criminal law provides for offences against society as a whole and is primarily a punitive system. Cases must be proved beyond reasonable doubt, the normal standard in criminal law. No compensation may be granted to injured employees. Prosecution will often result in a fine for the employer: though most are modest, there is no upper limit for cases brought in the Crown Court. The largest fine levied under the Health and Safety at Work Act was £750 000 for an incident at BP's Grangemouth Refinery in 1988 which resulted in three fatalities.

When a fatal accident has occurred, the Crown Prosecution Service may also bring a case for manslaughter. Despite there having been 3369 work related deaths reported in the past 10 years, only three employers have been convicted of manslaughter. The law in this area is very confused, prompting the Law Commission to propose a new general offence under this heading. Corporate liability has been held only in small companies where the "directing mind" is easily identifiable as one person. In a large business like P & O, that may be impossible. At Zeebrugge on 6 March 1987, 188 people died when the ferry *Herald of Free Enterprise* capsized. Charges failed because no single senior individual was found sufficiently at fault. Private prosecutions were brought after 51 people died when the pleasure cruiser *Marchioness* sank in 1989 and after the explosion on the oil rig Piper Alpha that killed 167 people. In both cases the actions failed.

Manslaughter cases for work related deaths

- The codirectors of a plastics company, Norman and David Holt, were prosecuted in 1988 after a worker had died from falling into a machine. This was the first individual prosecution of company directors for work related manslaughter—Norman Holt received a suspended sentence
- The managing director of OLL Ltd, Peter Kite, received the first immediate custodial sentence of two years. Four teenagers drowned during a canoeing trip across Lyme bay in 1993, and Kite was found in criminal neglect of his duty. The company was also found guilty of manslaughter and fined £60 000
- The trawler *Pescado* sank off Falmouth in 1991 with the loss of all six crew. The managing agent, Joseph O'Connor, was acquitted of manslaughter charges but found guilty of gross negligence, with a three year sentence, in 1996
- Jackson Transport (Ossett) Ltd and its director, Alan Jackson, currently face manslaughter charges after the death of an employee

---

Effect of European Commission directives

Evolution of health and safety legislation

Early, risk specific legislation
- Wool, Goat Hair and Camel Hair Regulations 1905
- Horsehair Regulations 1907
- Anthrax Prevention Act 1919
- Hides and Skins Regulations 1921
- Bakehouses Welfare Order 1927
- Biscuit Factories Welfare Order 1927
- Sugar Factories Welfare Order 1931
- Factories Act 1961
- Offices, Shops and Railway Premises Act 1963

1974-88: development of more general legislation
General umbrella statute heralding new era of health and safety legislation
- Health and Safety at Work Act 1974
A total of seven European directives bearing on health and safety had a strong influence on
- Control of Asbestos at Work Regulations 1987
- Control of Substances Hazardous to Health Regulations 1988
- Noise at Work Regulations 1989

Since 1988: modern domestic legislation based on risk assessment
More than 20 European directives have produced a deluge of regulations, notably the "framework" directive and its daughters in 1989 resulting in the "six pack"
- Management of Health and Safety at Work Regulations 1992
- Workplace (Health, Safety and Welfare) Regulations 1992
- Provision and Use of Work Equipment Regulations 1992
- Personal Protective Equipment Regulations 1992
- Display Screen Equipment Regulations 1992
- Manual Handling Operations Regulations 1992

The main statute regarding workplace health is the 1974 Health and Safety at Work Act. This is an umbrella statute giving general duties to provide, among others, a "safe place of work." This act replaced a mass of detailed, prescriptive legislation that had been enacted over many years, each statute addressing a specific risk.

Recent health and safety law has been driven by the European Commission. This legislation may take the form of articles (of the Treaty of Rome), effectively the constitution of the European Community. Directives are adopted by the council of ministers, and Britain, as a member state, is obliged to implement them by a certain date. Domestic legislation is generally enacted to fulfil the requirements of the directives. Should the regulations fail to do this, there may be the possibility of an appeal to the European Court.

Legal aspects

Levels of duty imposed on employers by health and safety legislation

- *Absolute*—As in some parts of the Factories Act: "Every moving part . . . shall be fenced"
- *Practicable*—Must be carried out if feasible, regardless of cost, as in some parts of the Noise at Work regulations
- *Reasonably practicable*—This applies to most of the general duties of the Health and Safety at Work Act. The health risks are balanced against the time, money, and effort required to reduce risk

---

The "six pack" of health and safety regulations that came into force in January 1993 arose from this source. This included the display screen regulations and the manual handling regulations. Like all modern regulations, they are based on the principle of risk assessment—the employer is required to address the risk posed by a workplace activity and produce suitable steps to reduce any substantial risks to an acceptable level. Approved codes of practice accompany regulations to guide employers in these deliberations. Although they are not legally binding, they constitute good practice.

Role of Health and Safety Executive

Guidance to doctors if a patient has a work related illness

- Write to patient's employer confirming the diagnosis. If condition falls under RIDDOR, the employer has responsibility to report it to appropriate authority (self employed patients must report such conditions themselves)
- To establish whether compensation may be payable, refer patient to DSS office for:
  Leaflet NI 2 (AUG 93) *If you have Industrial Disease*—Lists prescribed diseases and how to claim
  Leaflet NI 6 (Feb 96) *Industrial Diseases Disablement Benefit*—Gives details of other possible benefits
- If you or your patient need advice contact EMAS at local HSE office.
- If patient is considering a suit for negligence, this should be undertaken only by a solicitor experienced in such work. Trade unions will help their members pursue this possibility.

The 1974 Health and Safety at Work Act introduced both the Health and Safety Commission and the Health and Safety Executive (HSE), which have advisory and enforcement roles in industry. This includes the Employment Medical Advisory Service (EMAS), which employs doctors and nurses to advise both employers and employees on health and safety issues and appoints doctors to perform regular health surveillance as required by certain regulations (such as the Control of Lead at Work regulations).

The Health and Safety Executive has the power to enter and inspect workplaces. Inspectors may act informally, through advice, or issue improvement or prohibition notices. A prosecution may result in a fine. The average fine in the lower courts for health and safety offences was £2002 in 1994-5. Rarely, courts may order prison sentences for health and safety offences. A demolition job that failed to control the escape of asbestos resulted in a three month sentence for the owner of the company in January 1996, the first immediate prison sentence for such an offence. Two company directors received sentences of four months in April 1996 for failing to meet prohibition notices.

Employment law

The Employment Rights Act 1996 requires a written statement of terms and conditions of employment be given to each employee, forming the basis of the contract between employer and employed. The contract may also include implied terms. The act specifies duties on both parties, including the duty of employers to take reasonable care of the health and safety of the employees

---

There is a considerable body of legislation, both European and domestic, which affects employment. The Employment Rights Act 1996 which came into force on 22nd August 1996 consolidates all employees' rights into a single piece of legislation. The major pre-existing statute in this area, the 1978 Employment Protection (Consolidation) Act, is incorporated unchanged into the new Act and the Industrial Tribunals Act 1996, which similarly consolidates all aspects of law concerning Industrial and Employment Appeal Tribunals. Other primary and subordinate legislation relates to issues of discrimination, pay, and sick pay and are supported by various influential codes of practice such as those produced by the Advisory, Conciliation, and Arbitration Service (ACAS).

Dismissal
One of the most common problems arising in this area, which may involve occupational health physicians, is that of dismissal. Employees have a basic right under the act not to be unfairly dismissed (some groups do not enjoy this protection, such as self employed contractors). In general a qualifying period of two years employment is required before a complaint for unfair dismissal may be brought. Some types of unfair dismissal, notably certain grounds relating to health and safety, require no such period.

Potentially fair reasons for dismissal

1 Relating to capability ("skill, aptitude, health, or any other physical or mental quality") or qualifications ("any degree, diploma, or other academic, technical, or professional qualification")
2 Relating to conduct (behaviour at, or sometimes outside, the workplace)
3 Redundancy
4 If employee cannot continue to work without breach of statutory duty—such as after loss of driving licence
5 Some other substantial reason (SOSR) sufficient to justify dismissal

---

Dismissal occurs when the contract of employment is terminated by the employer, when a fixed term contract expires and is not renewed, or when an employee terminates the contract as a result of the employers' conduct. There are five potentially fair reasons for dismissal. The burden of proof lies with the employer to demonstrate a fair reason. An industrial tribunal will judge the circumstances of the case including elements such as the size, resources, consistency of behaviour, and procedural correctness of the employer—in deciding reasonableness.

Disability Discrimination Act 1995

The existing quota system in the Disabled Persons (Employment) Act 1944 has been repealed. Person registered as disabled under that act will be regarded as having a disability under the new act, initially for three years. A new National Disability Council will have an advisory role.

Most of the provisions of the new act came into effect on 2 December 1996, with new duties on employers to accommodate disabled people. It will be unlawful to treat anyone with a disability less favourably for reasons relating to that disability.

Disability is defined as "a physical or mental impairment that has substantial and long term adverse effect on the individual's ability to carry out normal day to day activities." Long term means longer than one year, and substantial is rather unhelpfully described in the code of practice as "more than minor."

Progressive conditions and conditions corrected in whole or part by treatment will be included. Employers are expected to modify workplaces and job design to make reasonable accommodations. These provisions apply both to job applicants and to those who suffer ill health or accident while in employment.

Lynock v Cereal Packaging [1988] IRLR 510

"When one is dealing with intermittent periods of illness each of which is unconnected, it seems to us to be impossible to give a reasonable prognosis or projection of the possibility of what might happen in the future."

Circumstances in which disclosure of confidential medical information may become necessary

1 By statute—such as notification of an infectious or occupational disease
2 In connection with judicial proceedings—a court or tribunal can order release of medical information
3 In the public interest, if failure to disclose might expose someone to risk of death or serious harm. In the 1976 American case of Tarasoff a university medical centre was told by a patient of his intentions to harm another student, who was not warned and was subsequently murdered. Her family sued successfully for negligence in failing to breach confidence
4 Patients have rights to their own medical notes, depending on format and circumstances, under the Data Protection Act 1984, the Access to Medical Reports Act 1988, and the Access to Health Records Act 1990

Key references

- Kloss D. *Occupational health law.* Oxford: Blackwell Law, 1994.
- Wikeley NJ. *Compensation for industrial disease.* Aldershot: Dartmouth, 1993.
- Judicial Studies Board. *Guidelines for the assessment of general damages in PI cases.* London: Blackstone Press, 1994.
- Kennedy I, Grubb A. *Medical law.* Sevenoaks: Butterworths, 1994.
- Brazier M. *Medicine, patients and the law.* London: Penguin, 1992.

Employees who are absent from work for reasons attributed to ill health often involve an occupational health physician. In dealing with these cases, it is important to differentiate between two situations—that of long term absence and the problem of persistent short term absence (or attendance). The first of these may give rise to fair dismissal on grounds of capability, which includes ill health and incompetence. The employer is expected to gather enough information to fully assess the situation and decide on a reasonable course of action. This will include a medical opinion. Confidentiality requires that the employer should not know details of the diagnosis but is entitled to ask:

- When might the employee recover?
- Will the employee be capable of returning to his or her former job?
- If not, what kind of restrictions upon capability are likely?

The physician giving an opinion must take steps to understand the requirements of the job and must have the employee's consent before assessing his or her medical condition for the purposes of the employer. Communication with others involved in clinical care, if appropriate, is also wise. The final decision on employment is a management rather than a medical decision, with the physician advising management in response to their questions. It is also important to appreciate that the cause of the ill health is irrelevant to the fairness of the dismissal; even if it is likely that the current employment has caused the ill health.

The problem of persistent short term absence is approached very differently by tribunals. Employers may view this as an attendance issue and take a more disciplinary line in managing it. The genuineness of the illness is not relevant—an employer is entitled to expect a reasonable level of attendance and may ultimately fairly dismiss on the grounds of "some other substantial reason." It is good practice (though not essential, depending on the case) to take medical advice as to whether there is any important underlying medical condition that may account for poor attendance. (If there is, the case might more properly be dealt with as a capability problem.) The situation was explained by the Employment Appeal Tribunal, which deals with appeals on matters of law arising from industrial tribunals, in the case of Lynock v Cereal Packaging.

A complaint of unfair dismissal is brought to an industrial tribunal within three months of the date of termination. The tribunal may order reinstatement (< 2% of cases), re-engagement, or compensation (which is limited, the maximum basic award being £6150).

Confidentiality

The duty of confidentiality upon any doctor is relative rather than absolute, and the legal basis of this duty remains unclear. There are circumstances in which disclosure of confidential medical information may become necessary.

Particular difficulties may arise for occupational health physicians, because of their employment by the company they advise. The position is actually quite clear; the physician is bound by the codes of his or her profession, and the employer cannot insist on any contractual terms that would require the physician to breach those codes. To do so would generate a contract which would be void. The occupational health physician should safeguard the confidentiality of all undertakings with patients/employees and their records in the same way as any other doctor.

The photograph of the 19th century foundry was reproduced with permission of Hulton Deutsch and the photograph of the Zeebrugge disaster was reproduced with permission of Rex Features.

INDEX

Index

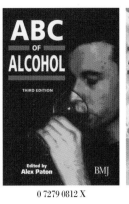
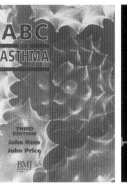
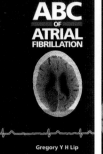
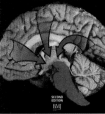
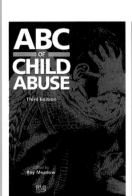
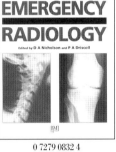
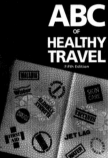
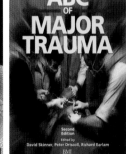
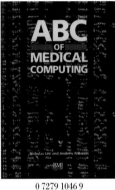
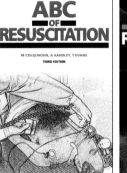
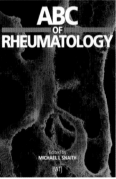
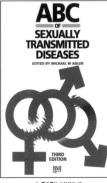
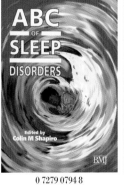
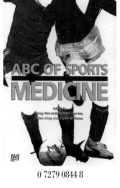
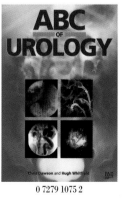